Mometrix

TEST PREPARATION

ACNPC®

Exam Secrets Study Guide

Dear Future Exam Success Story

First of all, **THANK YOU** for purchasing Mometrix study materials!

Second, congratulations! You are one of the few determined test-takers who are committed to doing whatever it takes to excel on your exam. **You have come to the right place.** We developed these study materials with one goal in mind: to deliver you the information you need in a format that's concise and easy to use.

In addition to optimizing your guide for the content of the test, we've outlined our recommended steps for breaking down the preparation process into small, attainable goals so you can make sure you stay on track.

We've also analyzed the entire test-taking process, identifying the most common pitfalls and showing how you can overcome them and be ready for any curveball the test throws you.

Standardized testing is one of the biggest obstacles on your road to success, which only increases the importance of doing well in the high-pressure, high-stakes environment of test day. Your results on this test could have a significant impact on your future, and this guide provides the information and practical advice to help you achieve your full potential on test day.

Your success is our success

We would love to hear from you! If you would like to share the story of your exam success or if you have any questions or comments in regard to our products, please contact us at **800-673-8175** or **support@mometrix.com**.

Thanks again for your business and we wish you continued success!

Sincerely,
The Mometrix Test Preparation Team

Need more help? Check out our flashcards at:
http://MometrixFlashcards.com/ACNPC

Written and edited by the Mometrix Exam Secrets Test Prep Team
Printed in the United States of America

TABLE OF CONTENTS

Introduction

Thank you for purchasing this resource! You have made the choice to prepare yourself for a test that could have a huge impact on your future, and this guide is designed to help you be fully ready for test day. Obviously, it's important to have a solid understanding of the test material, but you also need to be prepared for the unique environment and stressors of the test, so that you can perform to the best of your abilities.

For this purpose, the first section that appears in this guide is the **Secret Keys**. We've devoted countless hours to meticulously researching what works and what doesn't, and we've boiled down our findings to the five most impactful steps you can take to improve your performance on the test. We start at the beginning with study planning and move through the preparation process, all the way to the testing strategies that will help you get the most out of what you know when you're finally sitting in front of the test.

We recommend that you start preparing for your test as far in advance as possible. However, if you've bought this guide as a last-minute study resource and only have a few days before your test, we recommend that you skip over the first two Secret Keys since they address a long-term study plan.

If you struggle with **test anxiety**, we strongly encourage you to check out our recommendations for how you can overcome it. Test anxiety is a formidable foe, but it can be beaten, and we want to make sure you have the tools you need to defeat it.

Secret Key #1 – Plan Big, Study Small

There's a lot riding on your performance. If you want to ace this test, you're going to need to keep your skills sharp and the material fresh in your mind. You need a plan that lets you review everything you need to know while still fitting in your schedule. We'll break this strategy down into three categories.

Information Organization

Start with the information you already have: the official test outline. From this, you can make a complete list of all the concepts you need to cover before the test. Organize these concepts into groups that can be studied together, and create a list of any related vocabulary you need to learn so you can brush up on any difficult terms. You'll want to keep this vocabulary list handy once you actually start studying since you may need to add to it along the way.

Time Management

Once you have your set of study concepts, decide how to spread them out over the time you have left before the test. Break your study plan into small, clear goals so you have a manageable task for each day and know exactly what you're doing. Then just focus on one small step at a time. When you manage your time this way, you don't need to spend hours at a time studying. Studying a small block of content for a short period each day helps you retain information better and avoid stressing over how much you have left to do. You can relax knowing that you have a plan to cover everything in time. In order for this strategy to be effective though, you have to start studying early and stick to your schedule. Avoid the exhaustion and futility that comes from last-minute cramming!

Study Environment

The environment you study in has a big impact on your learning. Studying in a coffee shop, while probably more enjoyable, is not likely to be as fruitful as studying in a quiet room. It's important to keep distractions to a minimum. You're only planning to study for a short block of time, so make the most of it. Don't pause to check your phone or get up to find a snack. It's also important to **avoid multitasking**. Research has consistently shown that multitasking will make your studying dramatically less effective. Your study area should also be comfortable and well-lit so you don't have the distraction of straining your eyes or sitting on an uncomfortable chair.

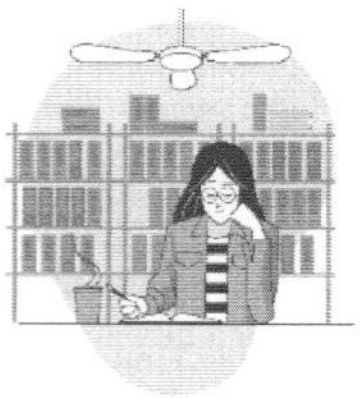

The time of day you study is also important. You want to be rested and alert. Don't wait until just before bedtime. Study when you'll be most likely to comprehend and remember. Even better, if you know what time of day your test will be, set that time aside for study. That way your brain will be used to working on that subject at that specific time and you'll have a better chance of recalling information.

Finally, it can be helpful to team up with others who are studying for the same test. Your actual studying should be done in as isolated an environment as possible, but the work of organizing the information and setting up the study plan can be divided up. In between study sessions, you can discuss with your teammates the concepts that you're all studying and quiz each other on the details. Just be sure that your teammates are as serious about the test as you are. If you find that your study time is being replaced with social time, you might need to find a new team.

Secret Key #2 – Make Your Studying Count

You're devoting a lot of time and effort to preparing for this test, so you want to be absolutely certain it will pay off. This means doing more than just reading the content and hoping you can remember it on test day. It's important to make every minute of study count. There are two main areas you can focus on to make your studying count.

Retention

It doesn't matter how much time you study if you can't remember the material. You need to make sure you are retaining the concepts. To check your retention of the information you're learning, try recalling it at later times with minimal prompting. Try carrying around flashcards and glance at one or two from time to time or ask a friend who's also studying for the test to quiz you.

To enhance your retention, look for ways to put the information into practice so that you can apply it rather than simply recalling it. If you're using the information in practical ways, it will be much easier to remember. Similarly, it helps to solidify a concept in your mind if you're not only reading it to yourself but also explaining it to someone else. Ask a friend to let you teach them about a concept you're a little shaky on (or speak aloud to an imaginary audience if necessary). As you try to summarize, define, give examples, and answer your friend's questions, you'll understand the concepts better and they will stay with you longer. Finally, step back for a big picture view and ask yourself how each piece of information fits with the whole subject. When you link the different concepts together and see them working together as a whole, it's easier to remember the individual components.

Finally, practice showing your work on any multi-step problems, even if you're just studying. Writing out each step you take to solve a problem will help solidify the process in your mind, and you'll be more likely to remember it during the test.

Modality

Modality simply refers to the means or method by which you study. Choosing a study modality that fits your own individual learning style is crucial. No two people learn best in exactly the same way, so it's important to know your strengths and use them to your advantage.

For example, if you learn best by visualization, focus on visualizing a concept in your mind and draw an image or a diagram. Try color-coding your notes, illustrating them, or creating symbols that will trigger your mind to recall a learned concept. If you learn best by hearing or discussing information, find a study partner who learns the same way or read aloud to yourself. Think about how to put the information in your own words. Imagine that you are giving a lecture on the topic and record yourself so you can listen to it later.

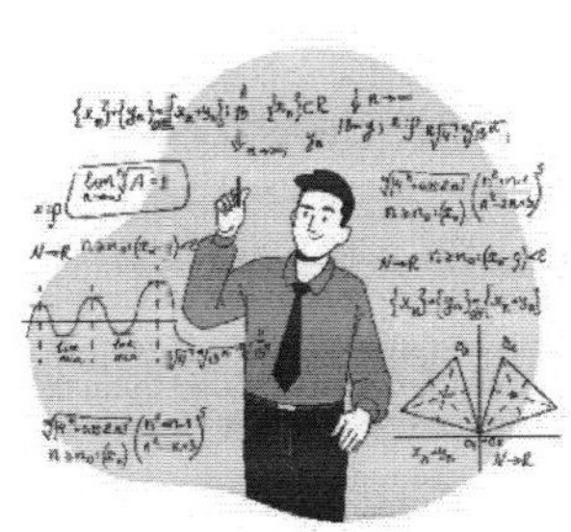

For any learning style, flashcards can be helpful. Organize the information so you can take advantage of spare moments to review. Underline key words or phrases. Use different colors for different categories. Mnemonic devices (such as creating a short list in which every item starts with the same letter) can also help with retention. Find what works best for you and use it to store the information in your mind most effectively and easily.

Secret Key #3 – Practice the Right Way

Your success on test day depends not only on how many hours you put into preparing, but also on whether you prepared the right way. It's good to check along the way to see if your studying is paying off. One of the most effective ways to do this is by taking practice tests to evaluate your progress. Practice tests are useful because they show exactly where you need to improve. Every time you take a practice test, pay special attention to these three groups of questions:

- The questions you got wrong
- The questions you had to guess on, even if you guessed right
- The questions you found difficult or slow to work through

This will show you exactly what your weak areas are, and where you need to devote more study time. Ask yourself why each of these questions gave you trouble. Was it because you didn't understand the material? Was it because you didn't remember the vocabulary? Do you need more repetitions on this type of question to build speed and confidence? Dig into those questions and figure out how you can strengthen your weak areas as you go back to review the material.

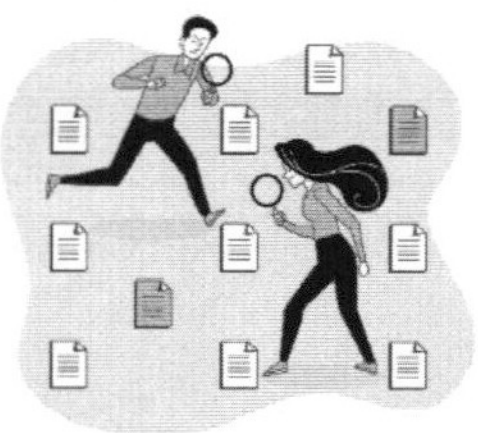

Additionally, many practice tests have a section explaining the answer choices. It can be tempting to read the explanation and think that you now have a good understanding of the concept. However, an explanation likely only covers part of the question's broader context. Even if the explanation makes perfect sense, **go back and investigate** every concept related to the question until you're positive you have a thorough understanding.

As you go along, keep in mind that the practice test is just that: practice. Memorizing these questions and answers will not be very helpful on the actual test because it is unlikely to have any of the same exact questions. If you only know the right answers to the sample questions, you won't be prepared for the real thing. **Study the concepts** until you understand them fully, and then you'll be able to answer any question that shows up on the test.

It's important to wait on the practice tests until you're ready. If you take a test on your first day of study, you may be overwhelmed by the amount of material covered and how much you need to learn. Work up to it gradually.

On test day, you'll need to be prepared for answering questions, managing your time, and using the test-taking strategies you've learned. It's a lot to balance, like a mental marathon that will have a big impact on your future. Like training for a marathon, you'll need to start slowly and work your way up. When test day arrives, you'll be ready.

Start with the strategies you've read in the first two Secret Keys—plan your course and study in the way that works best for you. If you have time, consider using multiple study resources to get different approaches to the same concepts. It can be helpful to see difficult concepts from more than one angle. Then find a good source for practice tests. Many times, the test website will suggest potential study resources or provide sample tests.

Practice Test Strategy

If you're able to find at least three practice tests, we recommend this strategy:

Untimed and Open-Book Practice

Take the first test with no time constraints and with your notes and study guide handy. Take your time and focus on applying the strategies you've learned.

Timed and Open-Book Practice

Take the second practice test open-book as well, but set a timer and practice pacing yourself to finish in time.

Timed and Closed-Book Practice

Take any other practice tests as if it were test day. Set a timer and put away your study materials. Sit at a table or desk in a quiet room, imagine yourself at the testing center, and answer questions as quickly and accurately as possible.

Keep repeating timed and closed-book tests on a regular basis until you run out of practice tests or it's time for the actual test. Your mind will be ready for the schedule and stress of test day, and you'll be able to focus on recalling the material you've learned.

Secret Key #4 – Pace Yourself

Once you're fully prepared for the material on the test, your biggest challenge on test day will be managing your time. Just knowing that the clock is ticking can make you panic even if you have plenty of time left. Work on pacing yourself so you can build confidence against the time constraints of the exam. Pacing is a difficult skill to master, especially in a high-pressure environment, so **practice is vital**.

Set time expectations for your pace based on how much time is available. For example, if a section has 60 questions and the time limit is 30 minutes, you know you have to average 30 seconds or less per question in order to answer them all. Although 30 seconds is the hard limit, set 25 seconds per question as your goal, so you reserve extra time to spend on harder questions. When you budget extra time for the harder questions, you no longer have any reason to stress when those questions take longer to answer.

Don't let this time expectation distract you from working through the test at a calm, steady pace, but keep it in mind so you don't spend too much time on any one question. Recognize that taking extra time on one question you don't understand may keep you from answering two that you do understand later in the test. If your time limit for a question is up and you're still not sure of the answer, mark it and move on, and come back to it later if the time and the test format allow. If the testing format doesn't allow you to return to earlier questions, just make an educated guess; then put it out of your mind and move on.

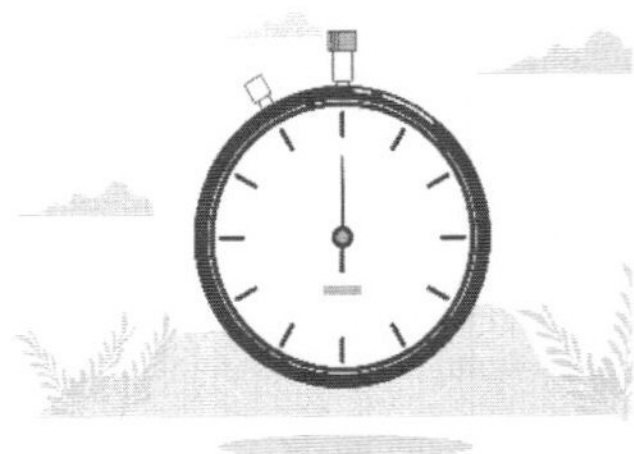

On the easier questions, be careful not to rush. It may seem wise to hurry through them so you have more time for the challenging ones, but it's not worth missing one if you know the concept and just didn't take the time to read the question fully. Work efficiently but make sure you understand the question and have looked at all of the answer choices, since more than one may seem right at first.

Even if you're paying attention to the time, you may find yourself a little behind at some point. You should speed up to get back on track, but do so wisely. Don't panic; just take a few seconds less on each question until you're caught up. Don't guess without thinking, but do look through the answer choices and eliminate any you know are wrong. If you can get down to two choices, it is often worthwhile to guess from those. Once you've chosen an answer, move on and don't dwell on any that you skipped or had to hurry through. If a question was taking too long, chances are it was one of the harder ones, so you weren't as likely to get it right anyway.

On the other hand, if you find yourself getting ahead of schedule, it may be beneficial to slow down a little. The more quickly you work, the more likely you are to make a careless mistake that will affect your score. You've budgeted time for each question, so don't be afraid to spend that time. Practice an efficient but careful pace to get the most out of the time you have.

Secret Key #5 – Have a Plan for Guessing

When you're taking the test, you may find yourself stuck on a question. Some of the answer choices seem better than others, but you don't see the one answer choice that is obviously correct. What do you do?

The scenario described above is very common, yet most test takers have not effectively prepared for it. Developing and practicing a plan for guessing may be one of the single most effective uses of your time as you get ready for the exam.

In developing your plan for guessing, there are three questions to address:

- When should you start the guessing process?
- How should you narrow down the choices?
- Which answer should you choose?

When to Start the Guessing Process

Unless your plan for guessing is to select C every time (which, despite its merits, is not what we recommend), you need to leave yourself enough time to apply your answer elimination strategies. Since you have a limited amount of time for each question, that means that if you're going to give yourself the best shot at guessing correctly, you have to decide quickly whether or not you will guess.

Of course, the best-case scenario is that you don't have to guess at all, so first, see if you can answer the question based on your knowledge of the subject and basic reasoning skills. Focus on the key words in the question and try to jog your memory of related topics. Give yourself a chance to bring the knowledge to mind, but once you realize that you don't have (or you can't access) the knowledge you need to answer the question, it's time to start the guessing process.

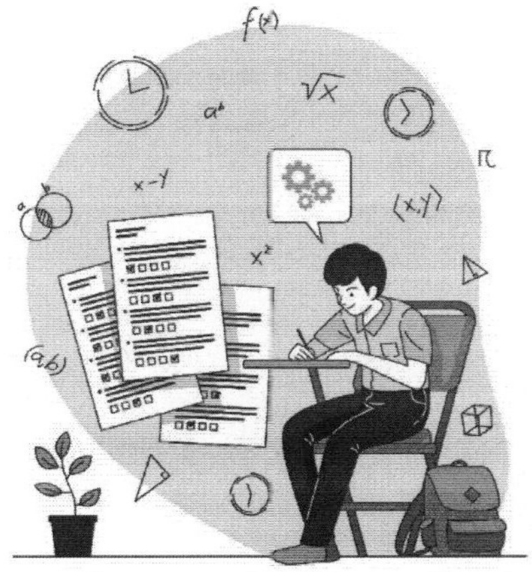

It's almost always better to start the guessing process too early than too late. It only takes a few seconds to remember something and answer the question from knowledge. Carefully eliminating wrong answer choices takes longer. Plus, going through the process of eliminating answer choices can actually help jog your memory.

Summary: Start the guessing process as soon as you decide that you can't answer the question based on your knowledge.

How to Narrow Down the Choices

The next chapter in this book (**Test-Taking Strategies**) includes a wide range of strategies for how to approach questions and how to look for answer choices to eliminate. You will definitely want to read those carefully, practice them, and figure out which ones work best for you. Here though, we're going to address a mindset rather than a particular strategy.

Your odds of guessing an answer correctly depend on how many options you are choosing from.

Number of options left	5	4	3	2	1
Odds of guessing correctly	20%	25%	33%	50%	100%

You can see from this chart just how valuable it is to be able to eliminate incorrect answers and make an educated guess, but there are two things that many test takers do that cause them to miss out on the benefits of guessing:

- Accidentally eliminating the correct answer
- Selecting an answer based on an impression

We'll look at the first one here, and the second one in the next section.

To avoid accidentally eliminating the correct answer, we recommend a thought exercise called **the $5 challenge**. In this challenge, you only eliminate an answer choice from contention if you are willing to bet $5 on it being wrong. Why $5? Five dollars is a small but not insignificant amount of money. It's an amount you could afford to lose but wouldn't want to throw away. And while losing $5 once might not hurt too much, doing it twenty times will set you back $100. In the same way, each small decision you make—eliminating a choice here, guessing on a question there—won't by itself impact your score very much, but when you put them all together, they can make a big difference. By holding each answer choice elimination decision to a higher standard, you can reduce the risk of accidentally eliminating the correct answer.

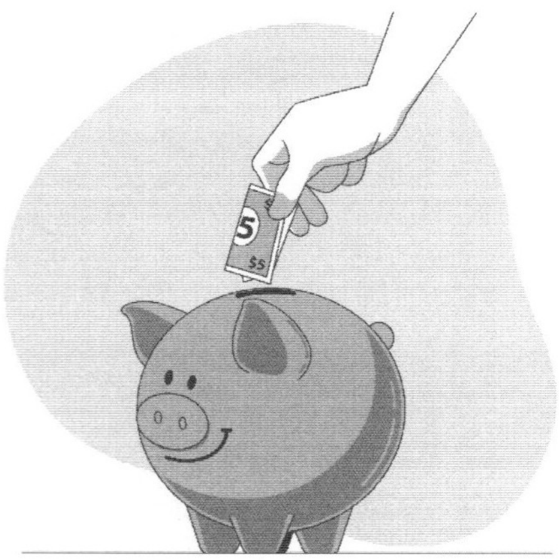

The $5 challenge can also be applied in a positive sense: If you are willing to bet $5 that an answer choice *is* correct, go ahead and mark it as correct.

Summary: Only eliminate an answer choice if you are willing to bet $5 that it is wrong.

Which Answer to Choose

You're taking the test. You've run into a hard question and decided you'll have to guess. You've eliminated all the answer choices you're willing to bet $5 on. Now you have to pick an answer. Why do we even need to talk about this? Why can't you just pick whichever one you feel like when the time comes?

The answer to these questions is that if you don't come into the test with a plan, you'll rely on your impression to select an answer choice, and if you do that, you risk falling into a trap. The test writers know that everyone who takes their test will be guessing on some of the questions, so they intentionally write wrong answer choices to seem plausible. You still have to pick an answer though, and if the wrong answer choices are designed to look right, how can you ever be sure that you're not falling for their trap? The best solution we've found to this dilemma is to take the decision out of your hands entirely. Here is the process we recommend:

Once you've eliminated any choices that you are confident (willing to bet $5) are wrong, select the first remaining choice as your answer.

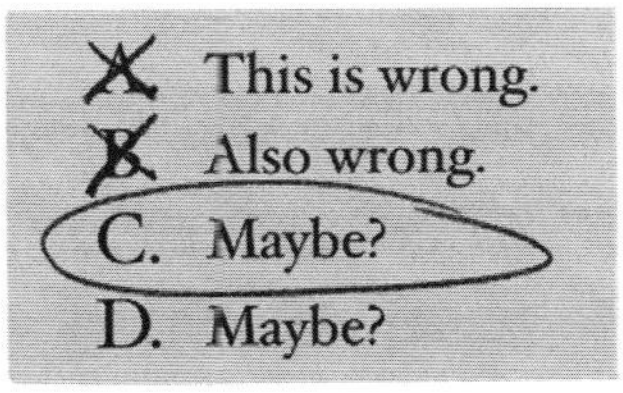

Whether you choose to select the first remaining choice, the second, or the last, the important thing is that you use some preselected standard. Using this approach guarantees that you will not be enticed into selecting an answer choice that looks right, because you are not basing your decision on how the answer choices look.

This is not meant to make you question your knowledge. Instead, it is to help you recognize the difference between your knowledge and your impressions. There's a huge difference between thinking an answer is right because of what you know, and thinking an answer is right because it looks or sounds like it should be right.

Summary: To ensure that your selection is appropriately random, make a predetermined selection from among all answer choices you have not eliminated.

Test-Taking Strategies

This section contains a list of test-taking strategies that you may find helpful as you work through the test. By taking what you know and applying logical thought, you can maximize your chances of answering any question correctly!

It is very important to realize that every question is different and every person is different: no single strategy will work on every question, and no single strategy will work for every person. That's why we've included all of them here, so you can try them out and determine which ones work best for different types of questions and which ones work best for you.

Question Strategies

☑ Read Carefully

Read the question and the answer choices carefully. Don't miss the question because you misread the terms. You have plenty of time to read each question thoroughly and make sure you understand what is being asked. Yet a happy medium must be attained, so don't waste too much time. You must read carefully and efficiently.

☑ Contextual Clues

Look for contextual clues. If the question includes a word you are not familiar with, look at the immediate context for some indication of what the word might mean. Contextual clues can often give you all the information you need to decipher the meaning of an unfamiliar word. Even if you can't determine the meaning, you may be able to narrow down the possibilities enough to make a solid guess at the answer to the question.

☑ Prefixes

If you're having trouble with a word in the question or answer choices, try dissecting it. Take advantage of every clue that the word might include. Prefixes can be a huge help. Usually, they allow you to determine a basic meaning. *Pre-* means before, *post-* means after, *pro-* is positive, *de-* is negative. From prefixes, you can get an idea of the general meaning of the word and try to put it into context.

☑ Hedge Words

Watch out for critical hedge words, such as *likely, may, can, often, almost, mostly, usually, generally, rarely*, and *sometimes*. Question writers insert these hedge phrases to cover every possibility. Often an answer choice will be wrong simply because it leaves no room for exception. Be on guard for answer choices that have definitive words such as *exactly* and *always*.

☑ Switchback Words

Stay alert for *switchbacks*. These are the words and phrases frequently used to alert you to shifts in thought. The most common switchback words are *but, although*, and *however*. Others include *nevertheless, on the other hand, even though, while, in spite of, despite*, and *regardless of*. Switchback words are important to catch because they can change the direction of the question or an answer choice.

☑ Face Value

When in doubt, use common sense. Accept the situation in the problem at face value. Don't read too much into it. These problems will not require you to make wild assumptions. If you have to go beyond creativity and warp time or space in order to have an answer choice fit the question, then you should move on and consider the other answer choices. These are normal problems rooted in reality. The applicable relationship or explanation may not be readily apparent, but it is there for you to figure out. Use your common sense to interpret anything that isn't clear.

Answer Choice Strategies

ANSWER SELECTION

The most thorough way to pick an answer choice is to identify and eliminate wrong answers until only one is left, then confirm it is the correct answer. Sometimes an answer choice may immediately seem right, but be careful. The test writers will usually put more than one reasonable answer choice on each question, so take a second to read all of them and make sure that the other choices are not equally obvious. As long as you have time left, it is better to read every answer choice than to pick the first one that looks right without checking the others.

ANSWER CHOICE FAMILIES

An answer choice family consists of two (in rare cases, three) answer choices that are very similar in construction and cannot all be true at the same time. If you see two answer choices that are direct opposites or parallels, one of them is usually the correct answer. For instance, if one answer choice says that quantity *x* increases and another either says that quantity *x* decreases (opposite) or says that quantity *y* increases (parallel), then those answer choices would fall into the same family. An answer choice that doesn't match the construction of the answer choice family is more likely to be incorrect. Most questions will not have answer choice families, but when they do appear, you should be prepared to recognize them.

ELIMINATE ANSWERS

Eliminate answer choices as soon as you realize they are wrong, but make sure you consider all possibilities. If you are eliminating answer choices and realize that the last one you are left with is also wrong, don't panic. Start over and consider each choice again. There may be something you missed the first time that you will realize on the second pass.

AVOID FACT TRAPS

Don't be distracted by an answer choice that is factually true but doesn't answer the question. You are looking for the choice that answers the question. Stay focused on what the question is asking for so you don't accidentally pick an answer that is true but incorrect. Always go back to the question and make sure the answer choice you've selected actually answers the question and is not merely a true statement.

EXTREME STATEMENTS

In general, you should avoid answers that put forth extreme actions as standard practice or proclaim controversial ideas as established fact. An answer choice that states the "process should be used in certain situations, if..." is much more likely to be correct than one that states the "process should be discontinued completely." The first is a calm rational statement and doesn't even make a definitive, uncompromising stance, using a hedge word *if* to provide wiggle room, whereas the second choice is far more extreme.

BENCHMARK

As you read through the answer choices and you come across one that seems to answer the question well, mentally select that answer choice. This is not your final answer, but it's the one that will help you evaluate the other answer choices. The one that you selected is your benchmark or standard for judging each of the other answer choices. Every other answer choice must be compared to your benchmark. That choice is correct until proven otherwise by another answer choice beating it. If you find a better answer, then that one becomes your new benchmark. Once you've decided that no other choice answers the question as well as your benchmark, you have your final answer.

☑ Predict the Answer

Before you even start looking at the answer choices, it is often best to try to predict the answer. When you come up with the answer on your own, it is easier to avoid distractions and traps because you will know exactly what to look for. The right answer choice is unlikely to be word-for-word what you came up with, but it should be a close match. Even if you are confident that you have the right answer, you should still take the time to read each option before moving on.

General Strategies

☑ Tough Questions

If you are stumped on a problem or it appears too hard or too difficult, don't waste time. Move on! Remember though, if you can quickly check for obviously incorrect answer choices, your chances of guessing correctly are greatly improved. Before you completely give up, at least try to knock out a couple of possible answers. Eliminate what you can and then guess at the remaining answer choices before moving on.

☑ Check Your Work

Since you will probably not know every term listed and the answer to every question, it is important that you get credit for the ones that you do know. Don't miss any questions through careless mistakes. If at all possible, try to take a second to look back over your answer selection and make sure you've selected the correct answer choice and haven't made a costly careless mistake (such as marking an answer choice that you didn't mean to mark). This quick double check should more than pay for itself in caught mistakes for the time it costs.

☑ Pace Yourself

It's easy to be overwhelmed when you're looking at a page full of questions; your mind is confused and full of random thoughts, and the clock is ticking down faster than you would like. Calm down and maintain the pace that you have set for yourself. Especially as you get down to the last few minutes of the test, don't let the small numbers on the clock make you panic. As long as you are on track by monitoring your pace, you are guaranteed to have time for each question.

☑ Don't Rush

It is very easy to make errors when you are in a hurry. Maintaining a fast pace in answering questions is pointless if it makes you miss questions that you would have gotten right otherwise. Test writers like to include distracting information and wrong answers that seem right. Taking a little extra time to avoid careless mistakes can make all the difference in your test score. Find a pace that allows you to be confident in the answers that you select.

☑ Keep Moving

Panicking will not help you pass the test, so do your best to stay calm and keep moving. Taking deep breaths and going through the answer elimination steps you practiced can help to break through a stress barrier and keep your pace.

Final Notes

The combination of a solid foundation of content knowledge and the confidence that comes from practicing your plan for applying that knowledge is the key to maximizing your performance on test day. As your foundation of content knowledge is built up and strengthened, you'll find that the strategies included in this chapter become more and more effective in helping you quickly sift through the distractions and traps of the test to isolate the correct answer.

Now that you're preparing to move forward into the test content chapters of this book, be sure to keep your goal in mind. As you read, think about how you will be able to apply this information on the test. If you've already seen sample questions for the test and you have an idea of the question format and style, try to come up with questions of your own that you can answer based on what you're reading. This will give you valuable practice applying your knowledge in the same ways you can expect to on test day.

Good luck and good studying!

Clinical Judgment

Cardiovascular

Heart Failure

Classes

Heart failure (HF) (formerly congestive heart failure) is a cardiac disease that includes disorders of contractions (systolic dysfunction) or filling (diastolic dysfunction) or both, and may include pulmonary, peripheral, or systemic edema. The most common causes are coronary artery disease, systemic or pulmonary hypertension, cardiomyopathy, and valvular disorders. The incidence of chronic heart failure correlates with age. There are two main types of HF: systolic and diastolic. HF is classified according to *symptoms* and prognosis:

- *Class I:* The patient is essentially asymptomatic during normal activities with no pulmonary congestion or peripheral hypotension. There is no restriction on activities, and prognosis is good.
- *Class II:* Symptoms appear with physical exertion but are usually absent at rest, resulting in some limitations of activities of daily living (ADLs). Slight pulmonary edema may be evident by basilar rales. Prognosis is good.
- *Class III:* Obvious limitations of ADLs and discomfort on any exertion. Prognosis is fair.
- *Class IV:* Symptoms at rest. Prognosis is poor.

Chronic heart failure develops more slowly with the myocardium damaged by lack of adequate oxygenation and nutrition, so that the myocardial cells begin to die. This creates areas of necrosis, which in turn stimulates the production of fibroblasts that replace cells with deposits of collagen, creating a fibrotic-resistant myocardium. Existing myocytes increase in size but lose strength. There is cardiac dilation and increasing vascular resistance (afterload).

Acute heart failure can occur with sudden onset, with the body attempting to compensate for circulatory malfunction by protecting blood flow to vital organs. There is an increase in the contractibility of the myocardium but peripheral vasoconstriction. Fluid and sodium are retained to control hypotension. However, the increased contractibility and heart rate increases the need for oxygen beyond that available, leading to a physiologic response that results in tissue necrosis, cardiotoxicity, pulmonary edema, and organ failure.

- Capillary hypertension decreases oncotic pressure and results in vasodilation and increased loss of fluid from the plasma to the interstitial fluid, resulting in pulmonary edema.
- Capillary hypotension results in increased oncotic pressure and pulls fluid back into the plasma, a result of shock.

Acute Heart Failure

Acute heart failure is characterized by impairment of gas exchange and decreased cardiac output because of changes in preload, contractibility, and heart rhythm. Patients may also suffer from anxiety, decreased activity tolerance, and disturbances in sleep patterns. Medical management is aimed at increasing cardiac function, providing support, and monitoring treatment.

Treatment may include:

- careful monitoring of fluid balance and weight to determine changes in fluid retention
- low-sodium diet
- restriction of activity

- medications may include diuretics, vasodilators, or ACE inhibitors to decrease the heart's workload; digoxin may be given to increase contractibility
- anticoagulant therapy if distended atria, enlarged ventricles, or atrial fibrillation occur, to decrease the danger of thromboembolia.

Patient education is an important component of heart failure management in order to prevent recurrence. The patient should be an active participant in planning care as the acute condition stabilizes.

Systolic Heart Failure

Systolic heart failure is the typical "left-sided" failure and reduces the amount of blood ejected from the ventricles during contraction (decreased ejection fraction), stimulating the sympathetic nervous system to produce epinephrine and norepinephrine to support the myocardium. However, this eventually causes down regulation in which beta and adrenergic receptor sites are destroyed, causing further myocardial damage. Because of reduced perfusion, the kidneys produce renin, which promotes angiotensin I, which is converted into angiotensin II, a vasoconstrictor, by the blood vessels. This in turns stimulates production of aldosterone, causing sodium and fluid retention. The end result of these processes is an increase in preload and afterload, increasing the workload on the heart, especially the ventricles. The heart muscle begins to lose contractibility and blood begins to pool in the ventricles, stretching the myocardium and enlarging the ventricles (ventricular remodeling). The heart compensates by thickening the muscle (hypertrophy) without an adequate increase in capillary blood supply because of the vasoconstriction of the coronary arteries, leading to ischemia.

Diastolic Heart Failure

Diastolic heart failure may be difficult to differentiate from systolic heart failure based on clinical symptoms, which are similar. With diastolic heart failure, the myocardium is unable to sufficiently relax to facilitate filling of the ventricles. This may be the end result of systolic heart failure as myocardial hypertrophy stiffens the muscles, and the causes are similar. Diastolic heart failure is more common in women older than 75 years of age. Typically, intracardiac pressures at rest are within normal range but increase markedly on exertion. Because the relaxation of the heart is delayed, the ventricles do not expand enough for the fill-volume, and the heart cannot increase stroke volume during exercise, so *symptoms* (dyspnea, fatigue, pulmonary edema) are often pronounced on exertion. Ejection fractions are usually greater than 40% to 50% with increase in left ventricular end-diastolic pressure (LVEDP) and decrease in left ventricular end-diastolic volume (LVEDV).

Acute Coronary Syndromes

Cardiogenic Shock

Cardiogenic shock usually results from MI damaging more than 40% of the left ventricle. *Diagnosis* includes ruling out other causes for the symptom:

- ECG: MI-related shock shows initial ST elevation and eventual Q waves; Clinical examination; Arterial blood gas analysis
- B-type natriuretic peptide (BNP) correlates with left ventricular end-diastolic pressure and pulmonary artery occlusion
- Echocardiogram shows impaired contractility of left ventricle
- Hemodynamic monitoring.
- *Treatment* includes stabilizing patient but may vary according to presenting symptoms and underlying cause:
- Supplemental oxygen and mechanical ventilation if in respiratory failure.
- IV access, arterial line, and urinary catheter.
- Nitroglycerine or morphine sulfate for chest pain.
- Aspirin (ASA) and heparin for MI.
- Inotropes for stabilization: dopamine, dobutamine.
- Diuretics as indicated.

- Thrombolytic therapy followed by intraaortic balloon counterpulsation and revascularization surgery by percutaneous coronary intervention or coronary bypass.
- Rapid transfer if necessary to facility equipped for invasive cardiac revascularization.

MYOCARDIAL INFARCTION

Myocardial infarction (MI) occurs when there is an imbalance between the heart's demand for oxygen and the supply. An MI is part of the continuum of acute coronary syndrome (ACS) and may occur after an episode of unstable angina caused by rupture of an atherosclerotic plaque and thrombosis associated with coronary artery spasm, but it may also result from vasoconstriction, acute blood loss, decreased oxygen, and ingestion of cocaine. Damage to the myocardium typically occurs in stages:

- Ischemia develops as oxygen levels fall, creating a zone of ischemia with viable cells.
- Cellular injury occurs to those cells surrounding the infarcted area in the zone of injury.
- Infarction with necrosis of tissue is the zone of infarction, where cells are destroyed and eventually replaced with scar tissue.

An MI is classified according to the extent of injury and necrosis, location, and the affected muscle layers.

TYPES OF MYOCARDIAL INFARCTION

Myocardial infarctions are classified according to their location and the extent of injury. Transmural myocardial infarction involves the full thickness of the heart (the endocardium, myocardium, and epicardium), often producing a series of Q waves on ECG. An MI most frequently damages the left ventricle and the septum, but the right ventricle may be damaged, depending upon the damaged area:

- *Anterior wall infarction* occurs with occlusion in the proximal left anterior descending artery, and may damage the left ventricle.
- *Left lateral wall infarction* occurs with occlusion of the circumflex coronary artery, often causing damage to anterior wall as well.
- *Inferior wall infarction* occurs with occlusion of the right coronary artery and causes conduction malfunctions.
- *Right ventricular infarction* occurs with occlusion of the proximal section of the right coronary artery and damages the right ventricle and the inferior wall.
- *Posterior wall infarction* occurs with occlusion in the right coronary artery or circumflex artery and may be difficult to diagnose.

CLINICAL MANIFESTATIONS

Clinical manifestations of MI may vary considerably, with men having the more "classic" symptom of sudden onset of crushing chest pain and women and those younger than 55 years of age presenting with atypical symptoms. Diabetic patients may have reduced sensation of pain because of neuropathy and may complain primarily of weakness. Elderly patients may also have neuropathic changes that reduce sensation of pain. More than half of all patients present with acute MIs with no prior symptoms of cardiovascular disease. *Symptoms* may include:

- angina with pain in chest that may radiate to neck or arms.
- palpitations
- hypertension or hypotension
- ECG changes (ST-segment and T-wave changes, tachycardia, bradycardia, and dysrhythmias)
- dyspnea
- pulmonary edema
- nausea and vomiting
- decreased urinary output
- paleness, skin cold and clammy

- diaphoresis
- dependent edema
- neurological/psychological disturbances: anxiety, light-headed, headache, visual abnormalities, slurred speech, and fear.

Diagnostic Procedures

Diagnosis of an MI includes a complete physical examination and patient and family history with assessment of risk factors. Assessment may include:

- *ECG* obtained immediately to monitor heart changes over time. Typical changes include T-wave inversion, elevation of ST segment, and abnormal Q waves.
- *Echocardiogram* to evaluate ventricular function.
- *Creatine kinase* (CK) and *isoenzyme* (MB): CK-MB (cardiac muscle) level increases within a few hours after onset of an MI, and peaks at about 24 hours (earlier with thrombolytic therapy or percutaneous transluminal coronary angioplasty [PTCA]).
- *Myoglobin* (heme protein that transports oxygen) found in both skeletal and cardiac muscles. Levels increase in 1 to 3 hours after an MI and peak within 12 hours. While an increase is not specific to an MI, a failure to increase can be used to rule out an MI.
- *Troponin* (protein in the myocardium) and its *isomers* (C, I, and T) regulate contraction and levels increase, in about the same time frame as CK-MB, but levels remain elevated for up to 3 weeks.

Acute Inflammatory Disease (Myocarditis)

Diagnosis of myocarditis depends upon the clinical picture, as there is no test specific for myocarditis, although the following tests may be done to verify the clinical diagnosis:

- Chest radiograph may indicate cardiomegaly or pulmonary edema.
- ECG may show nonspecific changes.
- Echocardiogram may indicate cardiomegaly and defects in functioning.
- Cardiac catheterization and cardiac biopsy will yield confirmation in 65% of cases, but not all of the heart muscle may be affected, so a negative finding does not rule out myocarditis.
- Viral cultures of nasopharynx and rectal may help to identify organism.
- Viral titers may increase as disease progresses.
- Polymerase chain reaction (PCR) of biopsy specimen may be most effective for diagnosis.

Treatment:

- As indicated for underlying cause (such as antibiotics).
- Restriction of activities.
- Careful monitoring for heart failure and medical treatment as indicated (e.g., diuretics, digoxin).
- Oxygen as needed to maintain normal oxygen saturation.
- IV gamma globulin for acute stage.

Peripheral Vascular Insufficiency

Peripheral vascular insufficiency involves both arterial and venous disease; however, venous disease is a chronic condition that rarely causes acute care crises. Peripheral arterial disease involves the aorta, its branches, arteries, and arterioles. Peripheral arterial disease often involves occlusion of the arteries of the lower extremities, resulting in severe pain and ischemia. The arteries most often affected by peripheral arterial disease are the femoral, the popliteal, the distal aorta, and the iliac arteries. The most common cause of arterial occlusion is atherosclerosis. *Symptoms* of peripheral arterial disease include:

- Intermittent claudication (a cramping pain while walking).
- Rest pain, a progression of intermittent claudication that includes pain even at rest. This requires catheter or surgical treatment to repair blockage.
- Tissue changes include thickening of nails, hair loss, and dry skin. Ulcerations may occur.

Acute occlusion, with pain, lack of pulses, decreased skin temperature, pallor, and loss of sensation and function. This requires immediate surgical intervention.

HYPERTENSION AND HYPERTENSIVE CRISIS

Blood pressure (BP) is the product of cardiac output and peripheral resistance, so hypertension can result from a change in cardiac output, peripheral resistance, or both. Normal blood pressure is less than 120 mm Hg systolic and less than 80 mm Hg diastolic. Hypertension is usually defined as systolic BP greater than 140 mm Hg systolic and greater than 90 mm Hg diastolic. Primary hypertension (90% to 95%) has no identified cause while secondary hypertension can be attributed to other disorders (such as renal disease, Cushing disease, or thyroid disease) or drug use, including corticosteroids. Most commonly, with essential hypertension, cardiac output is normal but peripheral resistance is increased. The following factors may be involved in causing hypertension:

- insufficient nephrons result in sodium retention and decreased filtration, causing increased fluid volume and increased preload
- stress triggers overactivity of the sympathetic nervous system, which causes increased contractibility, and/or renin-angiotensin excess, resulting in increased constriction and resistance
- genetic abnormalities may increase resistance
- obesity may result in hyperinsulinism that increases resistance through structural hypertrophy.

TYPES AND CAUSES

Hypertensive crises are marked elevations in blood pressure than can cause severe organ damage if left untreated. Hypertensive crises may be related to primary or secondary hypertension, which may result from kidney or endocrine disorders. Other diseases that may precipitate hypertensive crises include dissection of an aortic aneurysm, pulmonary edema, CNS disorders (subarachnoid hemorrhage, stroke), eclampsia, and failure to take medications properly. There are 2 classifications:

- *Hypertensive emergency* occurs when acute hypertension (1.5 times the 95th percentile), usually diastolic BP of greater than 120 mm Hg, must be treated immediately to lower blood pressure in order to prevent damage to vital organs, such as the heart, brain, or kidneys.
- *Hypertensive urgency* occurs when acute hypertension must be treated within a few hours but the vital organs are not in immediate danger.
- Blood pressure is lowered more slowly to avoid hypotension, ischemia of vital organs, or failure of autoregulation.
    - one-third reduction in 6 hours
    - one-third reduction in next 24 hours
    - one-third reduction over days 2 to 4

Treatment Options

Hypertensive crisis may be managed by a variety of different medications, depending upon the cause and whether the hypertension is an emergency or urgency. In some cases, medications may be combined. Patients with hypertensive emergency receive intravenous (IV) medications and oxygen. Medications include:

- Initial: Sodium nitroprusside (Nipride®) for fast-acting vasodilation.
- Short-acting beta-blockers (labetalol, esmolol) for dissecting aortic aneurysm.
- ACE inhibitors (enalapril) for heart failure.
- Nitroglycerine for chest pain.
- Dopamine-receptor agonist (fenoldopam) for renal disease to increase circulation to kidneys.
- Hydralazine for eclampsia.
- Calcium channel blocker (nicardipine) for CNS disorders.
- Enalaprilat and labetalol for CNS disorders.
- Alpha-blocker (phentolamine) for pheochromocytoma.
- Diuretics (e.g., furosemide, bumetanide) to reduce edema.
- Continuous monitoring of BP must be done. Observe the patient for hypotension caused by treatment. If the patient had a stroke, thrombolytic therapy (tissue plasminogen activator [tPA]) should not be given if the systolic BP is greater than 185 mm Hg and/or the diastolic BP is greater than 110 mm Hg.

Shock States

Perfusion

Assessment of perfusion can indicate venous or arterial abnormalities:

- *Venous refill time:* Begin with the patient lying supine for a few moments and then have the patient sit with the feet dependent. Observe the veins on the dorsum of the foot and count the seconds before normal filling. Venous occlusion is indicated with a time of greater than 20 seconds.
- *Capillary refill:* Grasp the toenail bed between the thumb and index finger and apply pressure for several seconds to cause blanching. Release the nail and count the seconds until the nail regains normal color. Arterial occlusion is indicated with a time of greater than 2 to 3 seconds. Check both feet and more than one nail bed.
- *Skin temperature:* Using the palm of the hand and fingers, gently palpate the skin, moving distally to proximally and comparing both legs. Arterial disease is indicated by decreased temperature (coolness) or a marked change from proximal to distal. Venous disease is indicated by increased temperature around the ankle.

Hypovolemic Shock

Hypovolemic shock occurs when there is inadequate intravascular fluid.

- The loss may be absolute because of an internal shifting of fluid or an external loss of fluid, as occurs with massive hemorrhage, thermal injuries, severe vomiting or diarrhea, and other injuries (such as ruptured spleen or dissecting arteries) that interfere with intravascular integrity.
- Hypovolemia may also be relative and related to vasodilation, increased capillary membrane permeability from sepsis or injuries, and decreased colloidal osmotic pressure that may occur with loss of sodium and some disorders such as hypopituitarism and cirrhosis.

Hypovolemic shock is classified according to the degree of fluid loss:

- Class I: less than 750 mL or 15% or less of total circulating blood volume (TCV)
- Class II: 750 to 1500 mL or 15% to 30% of TCV
- Class III: 1,500 to 2,000 mL or 30% to 40% of TCV
- Class IV: more than 2,000 mL or more than 40% of TCV.

Symptoms and Treatment

Hypovolemic shock occurs when the TCV of fluid decreases, leading to a fall in venous return that in turn causes a decrease in ventricular filling and preload, indicated by decreases in right atrial pressure (RAP) and pulmonary artery occlusion pressure (PAOP). This results in a decrease in stroke volume and cardiac output. This in turn causes generalized arterial vasoconstriction, increasing afterload (increased systemic vascular resistance), causing decreased tissue perfusion. *Symptoms* include:

- anxiety
- pallor
- cool and clammy skin
- delayed capillary refill
- cyanosis
- hypotension
- increasing respirations
- weak, thready pulse

Treatment is aimed at identifying and treating the cause of fluid loss and re-establishing an adequate intravascular volume of fluid through administration of blood, blood products, autotransfusion, colloids (such as plasma protein fraction), and/or crystalloids (such as normal saline). Oxygen may be given through intubation and ventilation if necessary. Medications may include a vasopressor, such as dopamine.

Cardiogenic Shock

Cardiogenic shock in adults most often is secondary to myocardial infarction damage that reduces the contractibility of the ventricles, interfering with the pumping mechanism of the heart, resulting in decreased oxygen perfusion. Cardiogenic shock has 3 characteristics:

- increased preload
- increased afterload
- decreased contractibility.

Together these result in a decreased cardiac output (less than 2.2 L/min) and an increase in systemic vascular resistance (SVR) to compensate and protect vital organs. This results in an increase of afterload in the left ventricle with increased need for oxygen. As the cardiac output continues to decrease, tissue perfusion decreases, coronary artery perfusion decreases, fluid backs up, and the left ventricle fails to adequately pump the blood, resulting in pulmonary edema and right ventricular failure. *Symptoms* include:

- hypotension with systolic BP less than 90 mm Hg.
- tachycardia greater than 100 beats/min with weak, thready pulse and dysrhythmias, decreased heart sounds
- chest pain, tachypnea, and basilar rales
- pallor, cool, moist skin

Septic Shock

Septic shock is caused by toxins produced by bacteria and cytokines that the body produces in response to severe infection, resulting in a complex syndrome of disorders. Symptoms are wide-ranging:

- Initial: hyper- or hypothermia, increased temperature (above 38ºC) with chills, tachycardia with increased pulse pressure, tachypnea, alterations in mental status (dullness), hypotension, hyperventilation with respiratory alkalosis ($PaCO_2$ 30 mm Hg or less), increased lactic acid, and unstable BP, and dehydration with increased urinary output
- Cardiovascular: myocardial depression and dysrhythmias
- Respiratory: acute respiratory distress syndrome (ARDS)

- Renal: acute renal failure (ARF) with decreased urinary output and increased BUN.
- Hepatic: jaundice and liver dysfunction with increase in transaminase, alkaline phosphatase, and bilirubin
- Hematologic: mild or severe blood loss (from mucosal ulcerations), neutropenia or neutrophilia, decreased platelets, and DIC
- Endocrine: hyperglycemia, hypoglycemia (rare)
- Skin: cellulitis, erysipelas, and fasciitis, acrocyanotic and necrotic peripheral lesions.

Septic shock is caused by toxins produced by bacteria and cytokines that the body produces in response to severe infection, resulting in a complex syndrome of disorders. Symptoms are wide-ranging:

- Initial: hyper- or hypothermia, increased temperature (above 38ºC) with chills, tachycardia with increased pulse pressure, tachypnea, alterations in mental status (dullness), hypotension, hyperventilation with respiratory alkalosis ($PaCO_2$ 30 mm Hg or less), increased lactic acid, and unstable BP, and dehydration with increased urinary output
- Cardiovascular: myocardial depression and dysrhythmias
- Respiratory: acute respiratory distress syndrome (ARDS)
- Renal: acute renal failure (ARF) with decreased urinary output and increased BUN.
- Hepatic: jaundice and liver dysfunction with increase in transaminase, alkaline phosphatase, and bilirubin
- Hematologic: mild or severe blood loss (from mucosal ulcerations), neutropenia or neutrophilia, decreased platelets, and DIC
- Endocrine: hyperglycemia, hypoglycemia (rare)
- Skin: cellulitis, erysipelas, and fasciitis, acrocyanotic and necrotic peripheral lesions.

Peripheral Arterial and Venous Disease

Arterial and Venous Insufficiency

Characteristics That Distinguish Arterial from Venous Insufficiency

Characteristic	Arterial	Venous
Type of pain	Ranges from intermittent claudication to severe and constant.	Aching and cramping.
Pulses	Weak or absent.	Present.
Skin of extremity	Rubor on dependency but pallor of foot on elevation.	Brownish discoloration around ankles and anterior tibial area.
	Skin pale, shiny, and cool with loss of hair on toes and foot.	
	Nails thick and ridged.	
Ulcers	Pain, deep, circular, often necrotic ulcers on toe tips, toe webs, heels, or other pressure areas.	Varying degrees of pain in superficial, irregular ulcers on medial or lateral malleolus and sometimes the anterior tibial area.
Extremity edema	Minimal.	Moderate to severe.

Peripheral Arterial Disease

Evaluation of the **pulses** of the lower extremities is an important part of assessment for peripheral arterial disease.

- Pulses should be first evaluated with the patient in supine position and then again with the legs dependent, checking bilaterally and proximally to distally to determine if intensity of pulse decreases distally. Pedal pulses should be examined at both the posterior tibialis and the dorsalis pedis. The pulse should be evaluated as to the rate, rhythm, and intensity, which is usually graded on a 0 to 4 scale:
    - 0 – pulse absent
    - 1 – weak, difficult to palpate
    - 2 – normal as expected
    - 3 – full
    - 4 – strong and bounding
- Pulses may be palpable or absent with peripheral arterial disease. Absence of pulse on both palpation and Doppler probe does indicate peripheral arterial disease.
- Bruits may be noted by auscultating over major arteries, such as femoral, popliteal, peroneal, and dorsalis pedis, and indicate peripheral arterial disease.

Venous Thromboembolism

Venous thromboembolism (VTE) is a condition that includes both deep vein thrombosis (DVT) and pulmonary emboli (PE). VTE may be precipitated by invasive procedures, lack of mobility, and inflammation, so it is a common complication in acute/critical care units. Virchow's triad comprises common risk factors: blood stasis, injury to endothelium, and hypercoagulability. Some patients may be initially asymptomatic, but *symptoms* may include:

- aching or throbbing pain
- positive Homan sign (pain in calf when foot is dorsiflexed)
- erythema and edema
- dilation of vessels
- cyanosis

Diagnosis may be made by ultrasound and/or D-dimer test, which test the serum for cross-linked fibrin derivatives. Computerized tomography (CT) scan, pulmonary angiogram, and ventilation-perfusion lung scan may be used to diagnose pulmonary emboli. Prophylaxis is very important, but once diagnosed, *treatment* involves bed rest, elevation of affected limb, anticoagulation therapy, and analgesics. Elastic stockings are worn when patient begins ambulating.

Interventions

The goals of management for arterial insufficiency and ulcers are to improve perfusion and save the limb, but lifestyle changes and medications may be insufficient. There are a number of indications for surgical intervention:

- Poor healing prognosis includes those with ankle-brachial index (ABI) less than 0.5 because their perfusion is severely compromised.
- Failure to respond to conservative treatment (medications and lifestyle changes) even with an ABI greater than 0.5.

- Intolerable pain, such as with severe intermittent claudication, that is incapacitating and limits the patient's ability to work or carry out activities. Rest pain is an indication that medical treatment is insufficient.
- Limb-threatening condition, such as severe ischemia with increasing pain at rest, infection, and/or gangrene. Infection can cause a wound to deteriorate rapidly.

Surgical intervention is indicated only for those patients with patent distal vessels as demonstrated by radiologic imaging procedures.

Pharmacologic to Maximize Perfusion

The primary focus of pharmacologic measures to maximize perfusion is to reduce the risk of thromboses:

- *Antiplatelet agents*, such as aspirin, ticlopidine (Ticlid®), and clopidogrel (Plavix®), which interfere with the function of the plasma membrane, interfering with clotting. These agents are ineffective to treat clots but prevent clot formation.
- *Vasodilators* may divert blood from ischemic areas, but some may be indicated, such as cilostazol, which dilates arteries and decreases clotting, and is used for control of intermittent claudication.
- *Antihyperlipidemic agents*, such as simvastatin and cholestyramine, slow progression of atherosclerosis.
- *Hemorheologic agents*, such as pentoxifylline, reduce fibrinogen, reducing blood viscosity and rigidity of erythrocytes; however, clinical studies show limited benefit. It may be used for intermittent claudication.
- *Analgesics* may be necessary to improve quality of life. Opioids may be needed in some cases.
- *Thrombolytics* may be injected into a blocked artery under angiography to dissolve clots.
- *Anticoagulants*, such as warfarin and enoxaparin, prevent blood clots from forming.

Dysrhythmias and Conduction Defects

Ventricle Septal Defect

Ventricular septal defect is an abnormal opening in the septum between the right and left ventricles. In children, the defect is often congenital, although it may be related to infarction in the adult. If the opening is small, the child may be asymptomatic, but larger openings can result in a left to right shunt because of higher pressure in the left ventricle. This shunting increases over 6 weeks after birth with symptoms becoming more evident. In some children, the defect may close within a few years, but in others it may persist into adulthood when symptoms become more evident. *Symptoms* may include signs of congestive heart failure with peripheral edema. About 10% of those with ventricular septal defect develop Eisenmenger's syndrome, characterized by increased pulmonary hypertension and right-sided heart failure with death often occurring by 40 years of age. Surgical repair includes pulmonary banding or cardiopulmonary bypass repair of the opening with suturing or a patch, depending upon the size.

Atrial Septal Defect

An atrial septal defect (ASD) is an abnormal opening in the septum between the right and left atria. It is often congenital, but may not be apparent until childhood or adulthood (in rare cases). Because the left atrium has higher pressure than the right atrium, some of the oxygenated blood returning from the lungs to the left atrium is shunted back to the right atrium where it is again returned to the lungs, displacing deoxygenated blood. *Symptoms* depend upon the degree of the defect but can include congestive heart failure, heart murmur, and increased risk for dysrhythmias and pulmonary vascular obstructive disease. Surgery may not be necessary for small defects, but larger defects require closure:

- Open-heart surgical repair may be done with general anesthesia and cardiopulmonary bypass (CPB).
- A closure device (Amplatzer septal occluder) is inserted through a minimally invasive cardiac catheter and placed across the atrial septal defect. This is an alternative procedure done with general anesthesia for children and local anesthesia and sedation for adults.

Cardiac Surgery

Surgical Options for Cardiac Valves

There are a number of different surgical options for repair of cardiac valves:

- *Valvotomy/Valvuloplasty* is usually done through cardiac catheterization. A valvotomy/valvuloplasty may involve releasing valve leaflet adhesions interfering with functioning of the valve. In balloon valvuloplasty, a catheter with an inflatable balloon is positioned in the stenotic valve and inflated and deflated a number of times to dilate the opening.
- *Aortic valve replacement* is an open-heart procedure with cardiopulmonary bypass. Aortic valves are tricuspid (3 leaflets) and repair is usually not possible, so defective valves must be replaced with either mechanical (metal, plastic, or pyrolytic carbon) or biological (porcine or bovine) xenografts.
- *Aortic homograft* uses part of a donor's aorta with the aortic valve attached to replace the recipient's faulty aortic valve and part of the ascending aorta.
- *Ross procedure* uses the patient's pulmonary artery with the pulmonary valve to replace the aortic valve and part of the aorta and then a donor graft is used to replace the pulmonary artery.

Coronary Artery Bypass Graft

Coronary artery bypass graft (CABG) is a surgical procedure for treatment of angina that does not respond to medical treatment, unstable angina, blockage of more than 60% in left main coronary artery, blockage of multiple coronary arteries including the proximal left anterior descending artery, left ventricular dysfunction, and previous unsuccessful percutaneous coronary interventions (PCIs). The surgery is performed through a midsternal incision that exposes the heart, which is chilled and placed on cardiopulmonary bypass with blood going from the right atrium to the machine and back to the body while the aorta is clamped to keep the surgical field free of blood. Bypass grafts are sutured into place to bypass areas of occluded coronary arteries. Grafts may be obtained from various sites:

- gastroepiploic artery
- internal mammary artery (commonly used and superior to saphenous vein but procedure is more time-consuming)
- radial artery
- saphenous vein (commonly used, especially for emergency procedures).

Acute Inflammatory Diseases

Acute Inflammatory Disease

Pericarditis is treated according to the cause and the type and extent of inflammation. Diagnostic procedures are similar to those for endocarditis and myocarditis. *Treatment* includes:

- Analgesics as indicated to control pain.
- Anti-inflammatory drugs, such as aspirin or ibuprofen, may be used to relieve discomfort and increase the rate of fluid reabsorption.
- Restriction of activity is necessary if cardiac function and output is impaired.
- Corticosteroids are used in some cases if there is no response to anti-inflammatory drugs.

Surgical intervention may include pericardiocentesis, which is removing fluid from the pericardial sac in order to relieve increasing pressure and to diagnose the causative agent. In some cases, a small opening may be made into the pericardium to allow continuous drainage of exudate into the chest cavity. In severe cases, the outer layer of the pericardium may need to be removed if it is preventing functioning of the ventricles.

Clinical symptoms of endocarditis usually relate to the response to infection, the underlying heart disease, emboli, or immunological response. Typical *symptoms* include:

- slow onset with unexplained low-grade and often intermittent fever
- anorexia and weight loss, difficulty feeding.
- general lassitude and malaise
- splenomegaly (in 60%) and hepatomegaly
- anemia (present in almost all patients)
- sudden aortic valve insufficiency or mitral valve insufficiency
- cyanosis with clubbing of fingers
- embolism of other body organs (brain, liver, bones)
- congestive heart failure
- dysrhythmias, new or change in heart murmur
- immunological responses:
- Janeway lesions: painless areas of hemorrhage on palms of hands and soles of feet
- splinter hemorrhages: thin, brown-black lines on nails of fingers and toes
- petechiae on oral mucous membranes, as well as hands and trunk
- Roth spots: hemorrhagic lesions on the retina caused by emboli on nerve fibers
- glomerulonephritis with hematuria found on microscopy.

Diagnosis and Treatment

Diagnosis of endocarditis is made on the basis of clinical presentation and diagnostic procedures that may include:

- Blood cultures should be done with 3 sets for both aerobic and anaerobic bacteria. Diagnosis is definitive if 2 cultures are positive, but a negative culture does not preclude bacterial endocarditis.
- Echocardiogram may identify vegetation on valves or increasing heart failure.
- Electrocardiogram (ECG) may demonstrate prolonged PR interval.
- Anemia (normochromic, normocytic).
- Elevated white cell count.
- Elevated erythrocyte sedimentation rate (ESR) and C-reactive protein (CRP).

Treatment includes general management of symptoms and the following:

- antimicrobials specific to the pathogenic organism, usually administered intravenously for 4 to 6 weeks
- surgical replacement of aortic and/or mitral valves may be necessary (in 30% to 40% of cases) if there is no response to treatment and/or after infection is controlled if there are severe symptoms related to valve damage.

Myocarditis

Myocarditis is inflammation of the cardiac myocardium (muscle tissue), usually triggered by a viral infection, such as influenza, Coxsackie virus, and HIV. Myocarditis can also be caused by bacteria, fungi, or parasites, or an allergic response to medications. In some cases, it is also a complication of endocarditis. It may also be triggered by chemotherapy drugs and some antibiotics. Myocarditis can result in dilation of the heart, development of thrombi on the heart walls (known as mural thrombi), and infiltration of blood cells around the coronary vessels and between muscle fibers, causing further degeneration of the muscle tissue. The heart may become enlarged and weak, as the ability to pump blood is impaired, leading to congestive heart failure. Symptoms depend upon the extent of damage but may include fatigue, dyspnea, pressure and discomfort in chest or epigastric area, and palpitations.

PERICARDITIS

Pericarditis is inflammation of the pericardial membrane that surrounds the heart. The outer fibrous pericardium is connective tissue that is continuous with the outer layers of the great vessels and serves to protect and anchor the heart. The inner serous pericardium has two layers separated with serous pericardial fluid to lubricate the heart and prevent friction. With pericarditis, the layers may become attached to each other (dry), or the serous fluid may be replaced by purulent material, calcifications, fibrinous material, or blood. Pericarditis is frequently associated with surgical repair of cardiac structural abnormalities, but it may also result from other systemic viral, bacterial, fungal, or parasitic infections, or may be caused by direct trauma. Some chronic connective tissue disorders, such as lupus erythematosus, may also cause pericarditis. Pericarditis is often accompanied by fever, dysrhythmia, poor appetite, irritability, malaise, and sharp, piercing chest pain.

ENDOCARDITIS

Endocarditis is an infection of the endothelial surface and valves of the heart. It is caused by invasion of the tissue by a pathogen, commonly streptococci staphylococci, enterococci, or pneumococci, as well as fungi and rickettsiae. Incidence is often hospital-acquired. Organisms enter the bloodstream from portals of entry (surgery, catheterization, IV drug abuse) and migrate to the heart, growing on the endothelial tissue and forming vegetations (verrucae), collagen deposits, and platelet thrombi. With endocarditis, the valves frequently become deformed, but the pathogenic agents may also invade other tissues, such as the chordae tendineae. The lesions may invade adjacent tissue and break off, becoming emboli. Endocarditis is associated with prolonged hospitalization, recent cardiac surgery (especially with synthetic grafts or valves), presence of pulmonary shunts, and invasive devices (such as central lines), and congenital heart disease as well as rheumatic heart disease with involvement of valves.

CARDIAC TAMPONADE

Cardiac tamponade occurs with pericardial effusion in which fluid accumulates in the pericardial sac, causing pressure against the heart. It may be a complication of trauma, pericarditis, cardiac surgery, or heart failure. About 50 mL of fluid normally circulates in the pericardial area to reduce friction, and a sudden increase in this volume can compress the heart, causing a number of cardiac responses:

- increased end-diastolic pressure in both ventricles
- decrease in venous return
- decrease in ventricular filling.

Symptoms may include a feeling of pressure or pain in the chest as well as dyspnea, and pulsus paradoxus greater than10 mm Hg (systolic blood pressure heard during exhalation but not during inhalation). Beck triad (increased central venous pressure with distended neck veins, muffled heart sounds, and hypotension) is commonly found. *Treatment* includes pericardiocentesis with large bore needle or surgical repair to control bleeding and relieve cardiac compression.

CARDIOMYOPATHIES

HYPERTROPHIC CARDIOMYOPATHY

Hypertrophic cardiomyopathy (also known as asymmetric septal hypertrophy) is a rare genetic and occasionally idiopathic disorder that is often undetected until adolescence when the increasing symptoms become noticeable. With hypertrophic cardiomyopathy, the heart mass and size increase, especially with thickness along the septum, resulting in smaller ventricular capacity so that the ventricles fill less efficiently and the atria have to work harder. This thickening may be asymmetrical. The disease may be nonobstructive or obstructive. The increased size of the septum may pull structures, such as the mitral valve, out of alignment, causing some obstruction of the flow of blood through the valve to the aorta (idiopathic hypertrophic subaortic stenosis). The changes in the ventricles may result in increasing diastolic abnormalities, although systolic function is usually normal or high. When diagnosed in young people, the disease is often more severe than in those who are diagnosed later in life.

Dilated Cardiomyopathy

Dilated cardiomyopathy, the most frequently occurring type of cardiomyopathy, occurs with an increase in the size of the ventricles (without a concomitant increase in hypertrophy of the ventricular muscle) as well as systolic dysfunction. The tissue loses elasticity and areas of myocardial cells become necrotic. This loss in elasticity results in less blood being ejected during ventricular systole so that during diastole, less blood is able to enter the partially filled ventricles. This results in both an increase in pressure at the end of diastole and also an increase in pulmonary pressure. As the ventricles stretch, the valves may be displaced, causing regurgitation. The poor blood flow can also cause thrombus formation and emboli. Many different conditions can cause dilated cardiomyopathy, including pregnancy, alcoholism, toxic compounds, autoimmune disease, and viral infections. Progress of the disease is often very slow, so diagnosis may be delayed until the disease is advanced and the patient suffers heart failure.

Restrictive Cardiomyopathy

Restrictive cardiomyopathy is the least common type of cardiomyopathy, but it is a common complication of heart transplants. However, if the heart function is very poor, one of the treatments for this disorder is heart transplantation. The condition may be idiopathic or secondary. The disease is often related to amyloidosis, a condition in which the protein amyloid is deposited in the cells, but many times the cause is unknown. While the heart may be almost normal in size, the ventricular walls become increasingly fibrotic and rigid so that the ventricles cannot relax and fill adequately during diastole. As the disease progresses, the ventricles also are unable to contract effectively, reducing blood flow, and increasing pulmonary and peripheral and systemic edema. Because there is no cure, early diagnosis and management of symptoms is important. The condition most commonly occurs in children but can affect young adults. Medical treatment includes the use of beta-blockers to allow the ventricles to fill more effectively.

Ruptured or Dissecting Aneurysm

Dissecting Aortic Aneurysms

A dissecting aortic aneurysm occurs when the wall of the aorta is torn and blood flows between the layers of the wall, dilating and weakening it until it risks rupture (which has a 90% mortality). Aortic aneurysms are more than twice as common in male patients than female patients, but female patients have a higher mortality rate, possibly because they are often older. Different classification systems are used to describe the type and degree of dissection. Common classifications include:

DeBakey classification uses anatomic location as the focal point:

- Type I begins in the ascending aorta but may spread to include the aortic arch and the descending aorta (60%). This is also considered a proximal lesion or Stanford type A.
- Type II is restricted to the ascending aorta (10% to 15%). This is also considered a proximal lesion or Stanford type A.
- Type III is restricted to the descending aorta (25% to 30%). This is considered a distal lesion or Stanford type B.

Type I and II are thoracic and type III is abdominal.

Treatment Options

Once a dissecting aortic aneurysm is identified, and the type is determined, both medical management and surgical repair may be indicated:

- Antihypertensives to reduce systolic BP such as beta-blockers (esmolol), or alpha/beta-adrenergic blocking agents (labetalol) to reduce force of blood as it leaves the ventricle to reduce pressure against aortic wall. IV vasodilators (sodium nitroprusside) may also be needed.
- Intubation and ventilation may be required if the patient is hemodynamically unstable.
- Analgesia/sedation to control anxiety and pain.

- Diagnostic tests, such as CT, MRI, transthoracic echocardiogram, and transesophageal echocardiograms may be needed.
- Type I and II are usually repaired surgically because of the danger of rupture and cardiac tamponade.
- Type III (abdominal) are often followed medically and surgery is delayed until aneurysm is greater than 5 cm, at which point either abdominal surgical repair or endoluminal stent may be done.

Pulmonary

Acute Respiratory Infections

Pneumonia

Pneumonia is inflammation of the lung parenchyma, filling the alveoli with exudate. It is common throughout childhood and adulthood. Pneumonia may be a primary disease or may occur secondary to another infection or disease, such as lung cancer. It may be caused by bacteria, viruses, parasites, or fungi. Common causes for community-acquired pneumonia (CAP) include:

- *Streptococcus pneumoniae*
- *Legionella species*
- *Haemophilus influenzae*
- *Staphylococcus aureus*
- *Mycoplasma pneumoniae,*
- *Viruses.*

Pneumonia may also be caused by chemical damage. Pneumonia is characterized by location:

- Lobar involves one or more lobes of the lungs. If lobes in both lungs are affected, it is referred to as "bilateral" or "double" pneumonia.
- Bronchial/lobular involves the terminal bronchioles and exudate can involve the adjacent lobules. Usually the pneumonia occurs in scattered patches throughout the lungs.
- Interstitial involves primarily the interstitium and alveoli where white blood cells and plasma fill the alveoli, generating inflammation and creating fibrotic tissue as the alveoli are destroyed.

There are a number of risk factors that can lead to aspiration pneumonitis/pneumonia:

- altered level of consciousness related to illness or sedation.
- diseases (Alzheimer or Parkinson)
- depression of gag, swallowing reflex
- intubation or feeding tubes
- ileus or gastric distention
- GI disorders, such as gastroesophageal reflux disorders (GERD).

With infants and small children, the most common causes of aspiration pneumonia are fluid or foods. Talcum powder used during diaper changes is also implicated. Toddlers and young children may aspirate lighter fluids or other hydrocarbon liquids. *Diagnosis* is based on clinical findings, ABGs showing hypoxemia, Infiltrates observed on x-ray, and increased WBC if infection is present. *Symptoms* are similar to other pneumonias, depending upon the site of inflammation: cough often with copious sputum, dyspnea, respiratory distress, cyanosis, tachycardia, and hypotension. *Treatment* includes:

- suctioning as needed to clear upper airway
- supplemental oxygen
- antibiotic therapy as indicated after 48 hours if symptoms not resolving symptomatic respiratory support.

Viral Pneumonia

Viral pneumonia is more common in adults than children, although the respiratory syncytial virus (RSV), which causes upper respiratory tract infections and bronchiolitis, can progress to pneumonia and is most commonly found in children 5 years of age or younger. A number of other viruses, such as adenoviruses, parainfluenza, cytomegalovirus, and coronavirus, may be implicated. The viruses invade the cells that line the airways and alveoli, causing death of the cells. *Symptoms* related to viral pneumonia are similar to those of bacterial pneumonia, although the onset is often slow, with pneumonia preceded by a respiratory tract infection that progressively worsens, with increasing cough, fever, dyspnea, cyanosis, and respiratory distress. There are few effective treatments for viral pneumonia, and one danger is that a viral pneumonia increases susceptibility to bacterial infection of the lungs. *Treatment* may include:

- rest and adequate fluids and nutrition
- antipyretics such as acetaminophen
- oxygen therapy with intubation and mechanical ventilation may be required in the presence of severe disease and respiratory compromise
- ribavirin aerosol is used for severe RSV disease and pneumonia.

Acute Bronchitis

Acute bronchitis is an inflammation of the bronchial tree in which swelling and exudate cause a partial obstruction that prevents the lung from fully inflating. Causes include viruses (most common), bacteria, yeasts and fungi, and noninfectious things, such as smoke or air pollutants. In adults, the most common viral triggers are influenza virus, adenovirus, and respiratory syncytial virus (RSV). *Symptoms* may include:

- dyspnea and tachypnea
- cyanosis
- heavy, productive, moist, or raspy cough.
- sputum clear, white, yellow, green, or bloody.
- localized crackling rales and expiratory high-pitched sibilant wheezes
- fever may or may not be present, but prolonged or high fever may indicate a bacterial infection.

Since most cases of acute bronchitis are caused by viruses and are self-limiting in 2 to 3 weeks, antibiotics are not helpful, but *treatment* may include:

- bronchial dilators (albuterol) to improve air exchange
- cough suppressant and/or expectorants to relieve cough
- antihistamines for those with allergic triggers
- antibiotics for bacterial infections

RSV

Bronchiolitis is inflammation of the bronchiolar level and is usually caused by the respiratory syncytial virus (RSV), although adenoviruses, parainfluenza, and *M. pneumoniae* have also been implicated. It is most common in infants and children between the ages of 2 months and 2 years and rarely occurs after that age. Most children who require hospitalization are infants younger than 6 months of age. The infection is usually seasonal and usually mild, although it can result in severe respiratory complications, so children should be observed carefully. *Symptoms* include dyspnea, a paroxysmal cough that is nonproductive, tachypnea, and wheezing. The infection is usually self-limiting and runs its course in 8 to 15 days but is highly contagious.

Treatment is usually symptomatic and includes:

- antipyretics such as acetaminophen
- oxygen therapy with intubation and mechanical ventilation may be required in the presence of severe disease and respiratory compromise ribavirin aerosol is used for severe disease.

Chronic Lung Disease

Asthma

An acute attack of asthma is precipitated by some stimulus, such as an antigen that triggers an allergic response, resulting in an inflammatory cascade that causes edema of the mucous membranes (swollen airway), contraction of smooth muscles (bronchospasm), increased mucus production (cough and obstruction), and hyperinflation of airways (decreased ventilation and shunting). Mast cells and T lymphocytes produce cytokines, which continue the inflammatory response through increased blood flow coupled with vasoconstriction and bronchoconstriction, resulting in fluid leakage from the vasculature. Epithelial cells and cilia are destroyed, exposing nerves and causing hypersensitivity. Sympathetic nervous system receptors in the bronchi stimulate bronchodilation. The 3 primary symptoms of asthma are cough, wheezing, and dyspnea. In cough-variant asthma, a severe cough may be the only symptom, at least initially.

Chronic Obstructive Lung Disease

Chronic obstructive lung disease (COPD) is a disease that causes limitations in airflow and may include both emphysema and chronic bronchitis, or more often a combination. The primary components to COPD include:

- progressive airflow limitation
- inflammatory response that causes a narrowing of the peripheral airways and thickening of the vessel walls of the pulmonary vasculature, exertional dyspnea and chronic cough.

Acute exacerbation can result in decompensation with increased hypoxemia (arterial oxygen saturation [SAO_2] less than 90% with tachycardia, tachypnea, cyanosis, and change in mental status) and hypercapnia (mental status change and hypopnea). Dyspnea and orthopnea are common symptoms. *Diagnosis* for severity includes pulmonary function tests, ABGs, chest x-ray (to rule out pneumonia or other complications), and echocardiogram.

Treatments include:

- oxygen with nasal cannula, facemask, Venturi mask, or non-rebreathing mask to elevate PAO_2 greater than 60 mm HG or SAO_2 greater than 90%
- beta-2 adrenergic agonists per nebulizer for bronchodilation
- anticholinergics: ipratropium bromide per metered inhaler
- corticosteroids: 60 to 180 mg/day for 7 to 14 days in decreasing doses, antibiotics for signs of infection
- assisted ventilation for muscle fatigue and respiratory acidosis.

Chronic Bronchitis

Chronic bronchitis is a pulmonary airway disease characterized by severe cough with sputum production for at least 2 consecutive years. Irritation of the airways (often from smoke or pollutants) causes an inflammatory response, increasing the number of mucus-secreting glands and goblet cells while ciliary function decreases so that the extra mucus plugs the airways. Additionally, the bronchial walls thicken and alveoli near the inflamed bronchioles become fibrotic, and alveolar macrophages cannot function properly, increasing susceptibility to infections. Chronic bronchitis is most common in those older than 45 years of age and occurs twice as frequently in women than men.

Symptoms include:

- persistent cough with increasing sputum
- dyspnea
- frequent respiratory tract infections.

Treatment includes:

- bronchodilators
- long-term continuous oxygen therapy or supplemental oxygen during exercise may be needed
- pulmonary rehabilitation to improve exercise and breathing
- antibiotics during infections
- corticosteroids may be used for acute episodes.

EMPHYSEMA

Emphysema, the primary component of COPD, is characterized by abnormal distention of air spaces at the ends of the terminal bronchioles, with destruction of alveolar walls so that there is less and less gaseous exchange and increasing dead space with resultant hypoxemia and hypercapnia and respiratory acidosis. The capillary bed is damaged as well, increasing pulmonary blood flow and raising pressure in the right atrium (cor pulmonale) and pulmonary artery, leading to cardiac failure. Complications include respiratory insufficiency and failure. There are 2 primary types of emphysema (and both forms may be present):

- *Centrilobular* (the most common form) involves the central portion of the respiratory lobule, with sparing of distal alveoli, and usually affects the upper lobes. Typical symptoms include abnormal ventilation-perfusion ratios, hypoxemia, hypercapnia, and polycythemia with right-sided heart failure.
- *Panlobular* involves enlargement of all air spaces, including the bronchiole, alveolar duct, and alveoli, but there is minimal inflammatory disease. Typical symptoms include hyperextended rigid barrel chest, marked dyspnea, weight loss, and active expiration.

ARDS/ALI

ARDS

Acute lung injury (ALI) comprises a syndrome of respiratory distress culminating in acute respiratory distress syndrome (ARDS), a rare complication of cardiac surgery. ALI and ARDS usually occur more than 24 hours postoperatively. ARDS is characterized by damage to the vascular endothelium and an increase in the permeability of the alveolar–capillary membrane when damage to the lung results from toxic substances (e.g., gastric fluids, bacteria, chemicals, toxins emitted by neutrophils as part of the inflammatory-mediated response); these substances reduce surfactant and cause pulmonary edema as the alveoli fill with blood and protein-rich fluid and then collapse (atelectasis). This decrease in surfactant also leads to decreased lung compliance (sometimes referred to as stiffening). The fluid in the alveoli becomes a medium for infection. Because there is neither adequate ventilation nor perfusion, the result is increasing hypoxemia and tachypnea as the body tries to compensate to maintain a normal partial pressure of carbon dioxide. Untreated, the condition results in respiratory failure, multiorgan failure, and death.

Patients presenting with **acute respiratory distress syndrome (ARDS)** may initially present with only mild tachypnea, but more serious *symptoms* develop as respiratory function becomes more compromised:

- crackling rales or wheezing may be heard throughout lungs
- decrease in pulmonary compliance (lung volume), referred to as "baby lung," results in increasing tachypnea with expiratory grunting
- cyanosis may develop with characteristic blue discoloration of lips and skin mottling
- hypotension and tachycardia may occur
- symptoms associated with volume overload are missing (third heart sound or jugular venous distention)
- respiratory alkalosis is often an early sign but is replaced as the disease progresses with hypercarbia and respiratory acidosis
- x-ray studies may be normal at first but then show diffuse infiltrates in both lungs, but the heart and vessels appear normal.

Management

The management of acute respiratory distress syndrome (ARDS involves providing adequate gas exchange and preventing further damage to the lung from forced ventilation. *Treatment* includes:

- Oxygen therapy by nasal prongs/cannula or mask may be sufficient in mild cases to maintain oxygen saturation above 90%. Oxygen should be administered at 100% because of the mismatch between ventilation (V) and perfusion (Q), which can result in hypoxia on position change.
- Endotracheal intubation may be needed if oxygen saturation falls or carbon dioxide levels rise.
- Mechanical ventilation with lower tidal volumes or high-frequency oscillatory ventilation to maintain oxygen saturation above 90%.
- Inhaled nitric oxide may be prescribed for pulmonary hypertension.
- Prophylactic antibiotics are not indicated.
- Steroids may increase survival rates if given later in treatment if ARDS has not resolved within a week.

Placing patient in prone position 18 to 24 hours/day with chest and pelvis supported and abdomen unsupported allows the diaphragm to move posteriorly, increasing functional residual capacity (FRC).

Respiratory Distress and Respiratory Failure

Pulmonary Hemorrhage

Pulmonary hemorrhage is an acute life-threatening injury that often results in death prior to arrival at the hospital; however, those presenting with traumatic pulmonary hemorrhage, as from a blunt or penetrating injury, requires immediate surgical repair. Even with immediate surgery, survival after serious injury to a major pulmonary vessel is rare. It is important that a large-bore IV be immediately inserted and fluid replacement begun while blood is typed and cross-matched. The patient should be evaluated for shock and treatment, including colloid solutions, crystalloids, or blood, provided as indicated. Pulmonary hemorrhage may result in hemothorax. In some cases, pneumothorax may also be present, resulting in mediastinal shift that increases the difficulty of identifying and repairing the bleeding vessel. If the patient is stabilized, computed tomography (CT) may provide accurate diagnosis to isolate the area of hemorrhage.

Obstructive Sleep Apnea

Obstructive sleep apnea results from passive collapse of the pharynx during sleep, often associated with a narrow or restricted upper airway (micrognathia, obesity, enlarged tonsils). It is most common in middle-aged, overweight men and is exacerbated by ingesting alcohol or sedative drugs before sleeping. *Symptoms* include daytime somnolence, headache, cognitive impairment, depression, personality changes, recent increase in weight, and impotence. Patients often snore loudly with cycles of breath cessation caused by apneic periods up to 60 seconds, occurring at least 30 times a night. ECG changes may indicate bradydysrhythmia during apnea and tachydysrhythmia when breathing resumes. *Diagnosis* is by polysomnography and evaluation of O_2 saturation during sleep. Laboratory findings include erythrocytosis. Thyroid function tests should be done to rule out hypothyroidism. *Treatment* includes weight loss, nasal continuous positive airway pressure [CPAP] at night, and surgical repair (uvulopalatopharyngoplasty and/or nasal septoplasty). Supplemental oxygen improves O_2 saturation but increases length of apneic periods and pharmacologic treatment is rarely helpful.

Narcolepsy

Narcolepsy is a sleep disorder characterized by three primary *symptoms*:

- Brief sudden episodes of falling asleep that can occur at any time and during any activity (usually 15 minutes or less).
- Loss of muscle tone (cataplexy), involving small muscle groups or generalized weakness, that causes the person to fall, slump, or freeze in place (may be confused with seizures).

- Sleep paralysis during which the person is conscious and alert but unable to move during the transition time between sleeping and waking.
- Abrupt rapid eye movement (REM) sleep resulting in hypnagogic auditory or visual hallucinations.

Treatments include:

- Dextroamphetamine sulfate 10 mg daily in AM. Side effects include headache, anxiety, and habituation.
- Modafinil 200 mg daily in AM to combat daytime drowsiness. Side effects less pronounced than for dextroamphetamine but may interfere with metabolism of other drugs, such as oral contraceptives.
- Imipramine 75 to 100 mg daily for cataplexy (not other narcoleptic symptoms)

STATUS ASTHMATICUS

Status asthmaticus is a severe acute attack of asthma that does not respond to conventional therapy, such as inhaled bronchodilators, and progresses to respiratory failure. The 3 primary *symptoms* of asthma are cough, wheezing, and dyspnea. In cough-variant asthma, a severe cough may be the only symptom, at least initially. The patient with status asthmaticus will often present in acute distress, nonresponsive to inhaled bronchodilators:

- Airway obstruction, sternal and intercostal retractions.
- Tachypnea and dyspnea, increasing cyanosis.
- Forced prolonged expirations.
- Cardiac decompensation with increased left ventricular afterload and increased pulmonary edema resulting from alveolar-capillary permeability. Hypoxia may trigger and increased pulmonary vascular resistance with increased right ventricular afterload.
- Pulsus paradoxus (decreased pulse on inspiration and increased on expiration) with extra beats on inspiration detected through auscultation but not detected radially. Blood pressure normally decreases slightly during inspiration, but this response is exaggerated.
- Hypoxemia (with impending respiratory failure).
- Hypocapnia followed by hypercapnia (with impending respiratory failure).
- Metabolic acidosis.

TREATMENT

Mechanical ventilation should be avoided if possible because of the danger of increased bronchospasm as well as barotrauma and decreased circulation. Aggressive medical management with beta-adrenergic agonists, corticosteroids, and anticholinergics should be tried prior to ventilation. However, the following are some absolute indications for the use of intubation and ventilation:

- cardiac and/or pulmonary arrest
- markedly depressed mental status (obtundation)
- severe hypoxia and/or apnea
- bradycardia.

There are a number of other indications that are evaluated on an individual basis and may be an indication for ventilation:

- exhaustion/ muscle fatigue from exertion of trying to breathe
- sharply diminished breath sounds and no audible wheezing
- pulse paradoxus greater than 20 to 40 mm Hg. If pulse paradoxus is absent, this is an indication of imminent respiratory arrest.
- PaO_2 less than 70 mm Hg on 100% oxygen
- deteriorating mental status
- dysphonia

- central cyanosis
- Increased hypercapnia
- metabolic/respiratory acidosis; pH less than 7.2.

ASPIRATIONS

FOREIGN BODY ASPIRATION

Foreign body aspiration can cause obstruction of the pharynx, larynx, or trachea, leading to acute dyspnea or asphyxiation, and the object may be drawn distally into the bronchial tree. With adults, most foreign bodies migrate more readily down the right bronchus. Infants and children, especially those weak or ill, are prone to aspiration of foreign substances (food, powder, secretions) or objects (dry nuts, candy, popcorn, toys). Sometimes the object causes swelling, ulceration, and general inflammation that hamper removal. *Symptoms* include:

- *Initial:* severe coughing, gagging, sternal retraction, wheezing. Objects in the larynx may cause inability to breathe or speak and lead to respiratory arrest. Objects in the bronchus cause cough, dyspnea, and wheezing.
- *Delayed*: hours, days, or weeks later, an undetected aspirant may cause an infection distal to the aspirated material. Symptoms depend on the area and extent of the infection.

Treatment includes:

- removal with laryngoscopy or bronchoscopy (rigid is often better than flexible)
- antibiotic therapy for secondary infection
- surgical bronchotomy (rare)
- symptomatic support

ACUTE PULMONARY EMBOLUS

ACUTE PULMONARY EMBOLISM

Acute pulmonary embolism occurs when a pulmonary artery or arteriole is blocked by a blood clot originating in the venous system or the right heart. While most pulmonary emboli are from thrombus formation, other causes may be air, fat, or septic embolus (from bacterial invasion of a thrombus). After cardiac surgery, most incidences are associated with deep venous thrombosis of the lower extremities. Other originating sites are the pelvic veins and the right atrium. Causes include stasis related to damage to the endothelial wall and changes in blood coagulation factors. Atrial fibrillation poses a serious risk because blood pools in the right atrium, forming clots that travel directly through the right ventricle to the lungs. The obstruction of the artery or arteriole causes an increase in alveolar dead space in which there is ventilation but impairment of gas exchange because of the ventilation–perfusion mismatching or intrapulmonary shunting. This results in hypoxia and the release of mediators that cause bronchoconstriction. Hypoxia leads to tachypnea which may present initially as respiratory alkalosis on early blood gas readings. In the case of severe hypoxia and systemic compromise that may ensue in later stages of a massive pulmonary embolism, a combination of metabolic and respiratory acidosis can occur. Metabolic acidosis occurs as a compensatory mechanism to the initial respiratory alkalosis, and in the case of systemic shut down and respiratory failure, respiratory acidosis can then result. If more than 50% of the vascular bed becomes excluded, pulmonary hypertension occurs.

SYMPTOMS AND DIAGNOSTIC TESTS

Clinical manifestations of **acute pulmonary embolism (PE)** vary, according to the size of the embolus and the area of occlusion.

Symptoms include the following:

- Dyspnea with tachypnea
- Tachycardia
- Anxiety and restlessness
- Chest pain
- Fever
- Rales
- Cough (sometimes with hemoptysis)
- Hemodynamic instability

The following diagnostic tests for **PE** are used:

- Arterial blood gas analysis may show hypoxemia (decreased partial pressure of oxygen), hypocarbia (decreased partial pressure of carbon dioxide), and respiratory alkalosis (increased pH) in early stages that may transition to metabolic and respiratory acidosis in the later stages of severe cases.
- D-dimer will show elevation with PE.
- Electrocardiogram may show sinus tachycardia or other abnormalities.
- Echocardiogram can show emboli in the central arteries and can assess the hemodynamic status of the right side of the heart.
- Chest x-ray is of minimal value.
- Spiral computed tomography may provide a definitive diagnosis.
- Ventilation–perfusion scintigraphy can confirm the diagnosis.
- Pulmonary angiograms also can confirm the diagnosis.

Medical management of PE starts with preventive measures for those at risk, including leg exercises, elastic compression stockings, and anticoagulation therapy (warfarin). Most pulmonary emboli present as medical emergencies, so the immediate task is to stabilize the patient.

Medical *treatment* may include:

- *oxygen* to relieve hypoxemia
- *IV* infusions
- *dobutamine* (Dobutrex®) or dopamine (Intropin®) to relieve hypotension
- cardiac monitoring for dysrhythmias
- *medications* as indicated: digitalis glycosides, diuretic, antiarrhythmics
- intubation and mechanical ventilation may be required
- *analgesia* (ex: morphine sulfate) or sedation to relieve anxiety
- Anticoagulation: prevents recurrence (but will not dissolve clots already present), including heparin and warfarin (Coumadin®).
- *placement of percutaneous venous filter* (Greenfield) in the inferior vena cava to prevent further emboli from entering the lungs may be done if anticoagulation therapy is contraindicated
- *thrombolytic therapy*, recombinant tissue-type plasminogen activator (rt-PA) or streptokinase, for those severely compromised, but these treatments have limited success and pose the danger of bleeding.

Air-Leak Syndromes

Air leak syndromes may result in significant respiratory distress. Leaks may occur spontaneously or secondary to some type of trauma (accidental, mechanical, iatrogenic) or disease. As pressure increases inside alveoli, the alveolar wall pulls away from the perivascular sheath and subsequent alveolar rupture allows air to follow the perivascular planes and flow into adjacent areas. There are two categories

- *Pneumothorax:*
  - Air in the pleural space causes a lung to collapse.
- *Barotrauma/volutrauma* with air in the interstitial space (usually resolve over time):
  - Pneumoperitoneum is air in the peritoneal area, including the abdomen and occasionally the scrotal sac of male infants.
  - Pneumomediastinum is air in the mediastinal area between the lungs.
  - Pneumopericardium is air in the pericardial sac that surrounds the heart.
  - Subcutaneous emphysema is air in the subcutaneous tissue planes of the chest wall.
  - Pulmonary interstitial emphysema (PIE) is air trapped in the interstitium between the alveoli.

Pneumothorax

Pneumothorax is a leak between the lung tissue and the chest wall so extraneous air is in the pleural space. Types include:

- *Spontaneous/Simple pneumothorax* is a breach of the parietal or visceral pleura, such as when an air-filled bleb on the lung surface ruptures or with a bronchopleural fistula without connection to outside air.
- *Traumatic pneumothorax* is a lacerating wound of the chest wall, such as a gunshot or knife wound. It can also result from invasive procedures, such as thoracentesis or lung biopsies or from barotrauma related to ventilation or chest surgery. Open pneumothorax occurs when air passes in and out, causing the lung to collapse, a sucking sound, and paradoxical movement of the chest wall with respirations.
- *Tension pneumothorax* is similar to traumatic open pneumothorax; however, the air can enter the pleural sac but cannot be expelled, causing a pronounced mediastinal shift to the unaffected side with severe compromise of cardiac and respiratory function.

Thoracic Surgery

Lung Repair and Surgery

Tracheal repair is rare but required for a variety of conditions:

- congenital stenosis
- complete tracheal rings
- postintubation stenosis
- trauma
- neoplasm
- tracheomalacia.

A variety of procedures are used for repair, depending upon the extent of involvement and other concomitant anomalies, such as pulmonary artery sling or bronchial abnormalities. Procedures include:

- Resection and anastomosis is effective if the involved area of the trachea is less than 30%, so it is used for short-segment stenosis.
- Slide tracheoplasty involves transecting the stenotic area and spatulating (making longitudinal cuts above and below the transection and then spreading the tissue to enlarge it) prior to reanastomosis. Slide tracheoplasty is used for long-segment stenosis with excellent results. This procedure uses the patient's own tissue, but follow-up bronchoscopies must be done to remove granulation tissue that tends to form.

Tracheal Surgery

Tracheal surgery includes:

- Pericardial patch creates an autologous graft to repair the trachea from a section of the pericardium. This procedure provides a good graft and rapid healing but requires cardiopulmonary bypass.
- Autologous graft may be created by using excised stenotic tracheal tissue for an anterior patch.
- Intraluminal stents may be used to support and prepare the trachea for further repair or to repair a failed tracheoplasty. A variety of stents, including the Dumon silastic stent, provide good support and are easily removed but cannot provide dilation. The metallic Palmaz stent is balloon-expandable and can be used to dilate a stenotic trachea, but it can be difficult to remove because of granulation tissue growing through the meshwork of the stent. However, this can be managed with repeated balloon dilations to provide pressure against the granulation tissue. Wire stents are permanent but require periodic dilation.

Lung Volume Reduction

Lung volume reduction surgery (LVRS) usually involves removing about 20% to 35% of lung tissue that is not functioning adequately in order to reduce the lung size so that the lungs work more effectively. This procedure is most commonly used with adult emphysematous COPD patients. In adults, surgery is usually bilateral; however, some patients are not candidates for bilateral surgery because of cardiac disease or emphysema affecting only one lung. Unilateral surgery has been shown to be effective. Surgical removal of part of the lung improves ventilation and gas exchange and does not require the immunosuppressive therapy required for lung transplantation. Studies have shown that those with low risk for the surgery and with emphysematous changes in the upper lobes can benefit from the surgery, but high-risk patients with more widespread emphysematous changes have increased mortality rates. The surgery may be done through an open-chest thoracotomy or through a less invasive video-assisted thoracotomy.

Pneumonectomy

Pneumonectomy is surgical removal of one of the lungs. There are 2 surgical procedures:

- *Simple*: removal of just the lung
- *Extrapleural*: removal not only of the lung but also part of the diaphragm on the affected side and the pericardium on that same side.

During the operative procedure, much care must be taken to prevent contamination of the remaining lung, including the use of bronchus blockers or prone position during surgery. Removal of the lung is indicated for a number of conditions:

- severe bronchiectasis from chronic suppurative pneumonia, resulting in dilation of terminal bronchioles
- severe hypoplasia
- unilateral lung destruction with pulmonary hypertension
- pulmonary hemorrhage
- lobar emphysema
- cancerous lesions (the most common reason for surgery)
- chronic pulmonary infections with destruction of lung tissue.

Because the lung capacity is reduced, persistent shortness of breath may occur with exertion even many months after surgery.

LOBECTOMY

- *Lobectomy* removes one or more lobes of a lung (which has 2 on the left and 3 on the right) and is usually done for lesions or trauma that is confined to one lobe, such as tubercular lesions, abscesses or cysts, cancer (usually non–small cell in early stages), traumatic injury, or bronchiectasis. Surgery is usually done through an open thoracotomy or video-assisted thoracotomy. Complications can include hemorrhage, postoperative infection with or without abscess formation, and pneumothorax. Usually 1 to 2 chest tubes are left in place in the immediate postsurgical period to remove air and/or fluid. Segmental resection removes a bronchovascular segment and is used for small lesions in the periphery, bronchiectasis, or congenital cysts or blebs.
- *Wedge resection* removes a small wedge-shapes portion of the lung tissue and is used for small peripheral lesions, granulomas, or blebs.
- *Bronchoplastic (sleeve) reconstruction* removes part of bronchus and lung tissue with reanastomosis of bronchus and is used for small lesions of the carina or bronchus.

TRACHEOSTOMY

Tracheostomy, surgical tracheal opening, may be utilized for mechanical ventilation. Tracheostomy tubes are inserted into the opening to provide a conduit and maintain the opening. Tracheostomy tubes are usually silastic or plastic, most lacking an inner cannula because they are nonadherent. The tube is secured with ties around the neck. Because the air entering the lungs through the tracheostomy bypasses the warming and moistening effects of the upper airway, air is humidified through a room humidifier or through delivery of humidified air through a special mask or mechanical ventilation. The patient with a tracheostomy must have continuous monitoring of vital signs and respiratory status to ensure patency of tracheostomy. Regular suctioning is needed, especially initially, to remove secretions:

- Suction catheter should be 50% the size of the tracheostomy tube to allow ventilation during suctioning.
- Vacuum pressure: 80 to 100 mm Hg.
- Catheter should only be inserted 0.5 cm or less beyond tube to avoid damage to tissues or perforation. Catheter should be inserted without suction and intermittent suction on withdrawal.

Review Video: Mechanical Ventilators
Visit mometrix.com/academy and enter code: 679637

PULMONARY HYPERTENSION

PULMONARY ARTERIAL HYPERTENSION

Pulmonary arterial hypertension (PAH) may involve multiple processes. Usually the pulmonary vasculature adjusts easily to accommodate blood volume from the right ventricle. If there is increased blood flow, the low resistance causes vasodilation and vice versa. However, sometimes the pulmonary vascular bed is damaged or obstructed, and this can impair the ability to handle changing volumes of blood. In that case, an increase in flow will increase the pulmonary arterial pressure, increasing pulmonary vascular resistance (PVR). This, in turn, increases pressure on the right ventricle (RV) with increased RV workload, and eventual RV hypertrophy with displacement of the intraventricular septum and tricuspid regurgitation. Over time, this leads to right heart failure and death. Pulmonary hypertension is usually diagnosed by right-sided heart catheterization, and is indicated by systolic pulmonary artery pressure greater than 30 mm Hg and mean pulmonary artery pressure greater than 25 mm Hg. Noninvasive testing may include echocardiogram to look for cardiac changes.

Medical treatment for pulmonary arterial hypertension (PAH) aims to identify and treat any underlying cardiac or pulmonary disease, control symptoms, and prevent complications:

- *Oxygen therapy* may be needed, especially supplemental oxygen during exercise.
- *Calcium channel blockers* may provide vasodilation for some patients.

- *Pulmonary vascular dilators,* such as IV epoprostenol (Flolan®), and subcutaneous treprostinil sodium (Remodulin®) and oral bosentan (Tracleer®), help to control symptoms and prolong life.
- *Anticoagulation*, with an anticoagulant such as warfarin, (Coumadin®) is an important part of therapy because of recurrent pulmonary emboli. Studies have shown that anticoagulation increases survival rates.
- *Diuretics*, such as furosemide (Lasix®), may be needed to relieve edema and restrict fluids, especially with right ventricular hypertrophy.

In some patients who cannot be managed adequately through medical treatment, a heart-lung transplant may be considered as the only effective treatment for long-term survival.

THORACIC TRAUMA

PULMONARY CONTUSION

Pulmonary contusion is the result of direct force to the lung, resulting in parenchymal injury and bleeding and edema that impact the capillary-alveoli juncture, resulting in intrapulmonary shunting as the alveoli and interstitium fill with fluid. Parenchymal injury reduces compliance and impairs ventilation. Diagnosis may be more difficult if other injuries, such as fractured ribs or pneumothorax, are also present because they may all contribute to respiratory distress. CT scans provide the best diagnostic tool.

Symptoms vary widely depending upon the degree of injury but may include:

- mild dyspnea
- severe progressive dyspnea
- hemoptysis
- acute respiratory failure.

Treatment varies according to the injury but can include:

- close monitoring of arterial blood gases and respiratory status
- supplemental oxygen
- intubation and mechanical ventilation with positive-end expiratory pressure (PEEP) for more severe respiratory distress
- fluid management and diuretics to control pulmonary edema
- respiratory physiotherapy to clear secretions.

FRACTURED RIBS

Fractured ribs are usually the result of severe trauma, such as blunt force from a motor vehicle accident or physical abuse. Underlying injuries should be expected according to the area of fractures:

- *Upper 2 ribs:* Injuries to trachea, bronchi, or great vessels.
- Right-sided ribs 8 to 12: Trauma to liver.
- Left-sided ribs 8 to 12: Trauma to spleen.

Pain, often localized or experienced on respirations or compression of chest way may be the primary symptom of rib fractures, resulting in shallow breathing that can lead to atelectasis or pneumonia.

Treatment is primarily supportive as rib fractures usually heal in about 6 weeks; however, preventing pulmonary complications often necessitates adequate pain control. Underlying injuries are treated according to the type and degree of injury:

- supplemental oxygen
- analgesia may include NSAIDs, intercostal nerve blocks, and narcotics
- pulmonary physiotherapy

Flail Chest

Flail chest is a more common injury in adults and older teens than children. It occurs when at least 3 adjacent ribs are fractured, both anteriorly and posteriorly, so that they float free of the rib cage. There may be variations, such as the sternum floating with ribs fractured on both sides. Flail chest results in a failure of the chest wall to support changes in intrathoracic pressure so that paradoxical respirations occur with the flail area contracting on inspiration and expanding on expiration. The lungs are not able to expand properly, decreasing ventilation, but the degree of respiratory distress may relate to injury to underlying structures more than the flail chest alone.

Treatment:

- analgesia for pain relief
- respiratory physiotherapy to prevent atelectasis
- mechanical ventilation is usually not indicated unless needed for underlying injuries
- surgical fixation is usually done only in those requiring thoracotomy for underlying injuries.

Hemothorax

Hemothorax occurs with bleeding into the pleural space, usually from major vascular injury such as tears in intercostal vessels, lacerations of great vessels, or trauma to lung parenchyma. A small bleed may be self-limiting and seal, but a tear in a large vessel can result in massive bleeding, followed quickly by hypovolemic shock. The pressure from the blood may result in inability of the lung to ventilate and a mediastinal shift. Often a hemothorax occurs with a pneumothorax, especially in severe chest trauma. Further symptoms include severe respiratory distress, decreased breath sounds, and dullness on auscultation. *Treatment* includes placement of a chest tube to drain the hemothorax, but with large volumes, the pressure may be preventing exsanguination, which can occur abruptly as the blood drains and pressure is reduced, so a large-bore IV line should be in place and typed and cross-matched blood immediately available prior to chest tube insertion. Autotransfusion may be used.

Pulmonary and Thoracic Trauma

The diagnostic procedures and tools used during assessment of pulmonary and thoracic trauma will vary according to the type and degree of injury, but may include:

- *Thorough physical examination* including cardiac and pulmonary status, assessing for any abnormalities.
- *Electrocardiogram* to assess for cardiac arrhythmias.
- *Chest x-ray* should be done for all those with injuries to check for fractures, pneumothorax, major injuries, and placement of intubation tubes. X-rays can be taken quickly and with portable equipment so they can be completed quickly during the initial assessment.
- *CT* may be indicated after initial assessment, especially if there is a possibility of damage to the parenchyma of the lungs.
- Oximetry and atrial blood gases as indicated.
- *12-lead electrocardiogram* may be needed if there are arrhythmias for more careful observation.
- *Echocardiogram* should be done if there is apparent cardiac damage.

Endocrine

Glycemic Disorders

Hyperglycemia

Hyperglycemia is elevation of serum glucose of at least 180 mg/dL, although symptoms may not be evident until the level reaches at least 270 mg/dL. The most common cause is diabetes mellitus (associated with decreased levels of insulin), but elevations of glucose may also be related to chronic pancreatitis, acromegaly,

Cushing syndrome, and adverse reactions to drugs, such as furosemide, glucocorticoids, growth hormone, oral contraceptives, and thiazides. Symptoms of hyperglycemia are similar to symptoms found in chronic diabetes and include ketoacidosis, polyuria, polydipsia, polyphagia, weight loss, and encephalopathy. Stress-related hyperglycemia is common after stroke and myocardial infarction and increases risk of mortality. Physiological stress related to infection may also increase glucose levels. Hyperglycemia can be treated with insulin and by treatment of the underlying cause or discontinuation of drug administration.

Hypoglycemia

Acute hypoglycemia (hyperinsulinism) may result from pancreatic islet tumors or hyperplasia, increasing insulin production, or from the use of insulin to control diabetes mellitus. Hyperinsulinism can cause damage to the central nervous and cardiopulmonary systems, interfering with functioning of the brain and causing neurological impairment. Causes may include:

- genetic defects in chromosome 11 (short arm)
- severe infections, such as gram-negative sepsis, endotoxic shock
- toxic ingestion of alcohol or drugs, such as salicylates
- too much insulin for body needs
- too little food or excessive exercise.

Symptoms include:

- blood glucose less than 50 to 60 mg/dL
- CNS: seizures, altered consciousness, lethargy, and poor feeding with vomiting, myoclonus, respiratory distress, diaphoresis, hypothermia, and cyanosis
- adrenergic system: diaphoresis, tremor, tachycardia, palpitation, hunger, and anxiety.

Treatment depends on underlying cause and includes:

- glucose/glucagon administration to elevate blood glucose levels
- diazoxide (Hyperstat®) to inhibit release of insulin
- somatostatin (Sandostatin®) to suppress insulin production
- careful monitoring.

Diabetes Mellitus

Diabetes mellitus is the most common metabolic disorder in children, affecting about 1.5 million children and adolescents with 70% to 85% with type 1 and the rest with type 2. More than 6% of adults have diabetes, but only two-thirds are diagnosed.

- **Type I:** Immune-mediated form with insufficient insulin production because of destruction of pancreatic beta cells.

Symptoms: Pronounced polyuria and polydipsia, short onset; may be overweight or recent weight loss, Ketoacidosis present on diagnosis

Treatment: Insulin as needed to control blood sugars, Glucose monitoring 1 to 4 times daily; Diet with carbohydrate control; Exercise

- **Type II:** Insulin resistant form with defect in insulin secretion.

Symptoms: Long onset; Obese with no weight loss or significant weight loss; Mild or absent polyuria and polydipsia; Ketoacidosis or glycosuria without ketonuria; Androgen-mediated problems such as hirsutism and acne (adolescents); Hypertension

Treatment: Diet and exercise, glucose monitoring, oral medications

> **Review Video: Diet, Exercise, and Medications for Diabetes**
> Visit mometrix.com/academy and enter code: 774388

Insulin

There are a number of different types of insulin with varying action times. Insulin is used to metabolize glucose for those whose pancreases do not produce insulin. People may need to take a combination of insulins (short- and long-acting) to maintain glucose control. Duration of action may vary according to the individual's metabolism, intake, and level of activity:

- *Humalog* (Lispro H) is a fast acting, short duration insulin that acts within 5 to 15 minutes, peaking between 45 and 90 minutes, and lasting 3 to 4 hours.
- *Regular* (R) is a relatively fast-acting, 30 minutes, insulin that peaks in 2 to 5 hours and last 5 to 8 hours.
- *NPH* (N) or *Lente* (L) insulin is intermediate acting with onset in 1 to 3 hours, peaking at 6 to 12 hours, and lasting 16 to 24 hours.
- *Ultralente* (U) is long-acting insulin with onset in 4 to 6 hours, peaking at 8 to 20 hours, and lasting 24 to 28 hours.
- *Combined NPH/Regular* (70/30 or 50/50) has an onset of 30 minutes, peaks at 7 to 12 hours, and lasts 16 to 24 hours.

Oral Hypoglycemic Agents

Oral hypoglycemic agents, also known as sulfonylureas, are used to treat type 2 diabetes mellitus. These drugs are derived from sulfonamide and bind to potassium channel receptors, preventing potassium efflux, allowing influx of calcium and release of insulin from pancreatic islets. They are effective in decreasing serum levels of glucagon and potentiating the production of insulin. There are both first-generation drugs and second-generation drugs, which have shorter half-lives and increased potency over first-generation. First-generation drugs include:

- *Acetohexamide* with half-life of 6 to 8 hours and duration of 12 to 18 hours.
- *Chlorpropamide* with half-life of 36 hours and duration of 60 hours.
- *Tolazamide* with half-life of 7 hours and duration of 12-14 hours.
- *Tolbutamide* with half-life of 4.5 to 6.5 hours and duration of 6 to 12 hours.

Second-generation drugs include:

- *Glipizide* with half-life of 4 hours and duration of 24 hours.
- *Glyburide* with half-life of 1.5 to 3 hours and duration of 24 hours.

HHNS

Hyperglycemic hyperosmolar nonketotic syndrome (HHNS) or hyperosmolar hyperglycemic state (HHS) occurs in persons without a history of diabetes or with mild type 2 diabetes but with insulin resistance resulting in persistent hyperglycemia, which causes osmotic diuresis. Fluid shift from intracellular to extracellular spaces to maintain osmotic equilibrium, but the increased glucosuria and dehydration results in hypernatremia and increased osmolarity. This condition is most common in those 50 to 70 years of age and often is precipitated by an acute illness, such as a stroke, medications such as thiazides, or dialysis treatments. HNNS differs from ketoacidosis because, while the insulin level is not adequate, it is high enough to prevent the breakdown of fat. *Symptoms* include:

- polyuria
- dehydration

- hypotension
- tachycardia
- blood glucose greater than 600 mg/dL
- serum osmolality greater than 350 mOsm/L
- increased blood urea nitrogen (BUN) and creatinine
- changes in mental status, seizures, hemiparesis.

Onset of acute symptoms usually occurs over a few days. *Treatment* is similar to that for ketoacidosis: Insulin and IV fluids and electrolytes.

KETOACIDOSIS

Ketoacidosis is a complication of diabetes mellitus. Inadequate production of insulin results in glucose being unavailable for metabolism, so lipolysis (breakdown of fat) produces free fatty acids as an alternate fuel source. Glycerol in both fat cells and the liver is converted to ketone bodies (beta-hydroxybutyric acid, acetoacetic acid, and acetone), which are used for cellular metabolism less efficiently than glucose. Excess ketone bodies are excreted in the urine (ketonuria) or exhalations. The ketone bodies lower serum pH, leading to ketoacidosis. *Symptoms* include:

- Kussmaul respirations: hyperventilation to eliminate buildup of carbon dioxide, associated with "ketone breath."
- Fluid imbalance, including loss of potassium and other electrolytes from cellular death, resulting in dehydration and diuresis with excess thirst.
- Cardiac arrhythmias, related to potassium loss, can lead to cardiac arrest.
- Hyperglycemia: blood glucose may vary (300 to 800 mg/dL).
- Normal values for fasting blood glucose: 60 to 100 mg/dL.

Treatment includes:

- insulin therapy by continuous infusion initially
- rehydration and electrolyte replacement

THYROID DISORDERS

HYPOTHYROIDISM

Hypothyroidism occurs when the thyroid produces inadequate levels of thyroid hormones. Conditions may range from mild to severe myxedema. There are a number of causes:

- chronic lymphocytic thyroiditis (Hashimoto thyroiditis)
- excessive treatment for hyperthyroidism
- atrophy of thyroid
- medications such as lithium or iodine compounds
- radiation to the area of the thyroid
- diseases that affect the thyroid such as scleroderma
- iodine imbalances.

Symptoms may include chronic fatigue, menstrual disturbances, hoarseness, subnormal temperature, low pulse rate, weight gain, thinning hair, and thickening skin. Some dementia may occur with advanced conditions. Clinical findings may include increased cholesterol with associated atherosclerosis and coronary artery disease. Myxedema may be characterized by changes in respiration with hypoventilation and CO_2 retention resulting in coma. *Treatment* involves hormone replacement with synthetic levothyroxine based on thyroid-stimulating hormone (TSH) levels, but this increases the oxygen demand of the body, so careful monitoring of cardiac status must be done during early treatment to avoid myocardial infarction while reaching euthyroid (normal) level.

Hyperthyroidism

Hyperthyroidism (thyrotoxicosis) usually results from excess production of thyroid hormones (Graves' disease) from immunoglobulins providing abnormal stimulation of the thyroid gland. Other causes include thyroiditis and excess thyroid medications. *Symptoms* vary and may be nonspecific, especially in elderly patients, and include:

- hyperexcitability
- tachycardia (90 to 160) and atrial fibrillation
- increased systolic (but not diastolic) BP
- poor heat tolerance, skin flushed, and diaphoretic
- dry skin and pruritus (especially in elderly patients)
- hand tremor, progressive muscular weakness
- exophthalmos (bulging eyes)
- increased appetite and intake but weight loss.

Treatment includes:

- Radioactive iodine to destroy the thyroid gland. Propranolol may be used to prevent thyroid storm. Thyroid hormones are given for resultant hypothyroidism.
- Antithyroid medications, such as methimazole (Propacil® or Tapazole®), to block conversion of T4 to T3.
- Surgical removal of thyroid is used if patients cannot tolerate other treatments or in special circumstances, such as large goiter. Usually one-sixth of the thyroid is left in place and antithyroid medications are given before surgery.

Review Video: Hyperthyroidism
Visit mometrix.com/academy and enter code: 923159

Thyrotoxic Storm

Thyrotoxic storm is a severe type of hyperthyroidism with sudden onset, precipitated by stress, such as injury or surgery, in those untreated or inadequately treated for hyperthyroidism. If not promptly diagnosed and treated, it is fatal. Incidence has decreased with the use of antithyroid medications but can still occur with medical emergencies or pregnancy.

Symptoms include:

- increase in symptoms of hyperthyroidism
- increased temperature higher than 38.5°C.
- tachycardia >than130 with atrial fibrillation and heart failure
- GI disorders, such as nausea, vomiting, diarrhea, and abdominal discomfort; altered mental status with delirium progressing to coma.
- Diagnostic findings are similar to hyperthyroidism, and include increased T3 uptake and decreased TSH.

Treatment includes:

- controlling production of thyroid hormone through antithyroid medications, such as propylthiouracil and methimazole
- inhibiting release of thyroid hormone: iodine therapy (lithium)
- controlling peripheral activity of thyroid hormone (propranolol)
- fluid and electrolyte replacement

- glucocorticoids, such as dexamethasone
- cooling blankets; treatment of arrhythmias (antiarrhythmics and anticoagulation

Adrenal Disorders

Addison's Disease

Adrenocortical insufficiency (Addison's disease) is caused by damage to the adrenal cortex, related to a variety of causes, such as autoimmune disease or genetic disorders, but it may relate to destructive lesions or neoplasms. Without treatment, the condition is life threatening.

Symptoms may be vague and the condition undiagnosed until 80% to 90% of the adrenal cortex has been destroyed:

- chronic weakness and fatigue
- abdominal distress with nausea and vomiting
- salt or licorice craving, resulting from deficiency of aldosterone
- pigmentary changes in skin and mucous membranes, hyperpigmentation
- hypotension
- hypoglycemia
- recurrent seizures (more common in children)

Treatment:

- Hormone replacement therapy with glucocorticoids (cortisol) and mineralocorticoids (aldosterone) may be taken orally or monthly parenteral injections or subcutaneous implantation of desoxycorticosterone acetate every 9 to12 months.
- During times of stress or illness, the demand for glucocorticoids may increase and dosages up to 3 times the normal dosage may be needed to prevent an acute crisis.

Acute Adrenal Insufficiency

Acute adrenal insufficiency (adrenal crisis) is a sudden, life-threatening condition resulting from an exacerbation of primary chronic adrenal insufficiency (Addison's disease), often precipitated by sepsis, surgical stress, adrenal hemorrhage related to septicemia, anticoagulation complications, and cortisone withdrawal related to decreased dose or inadequate dose to compensate for stress. Acute adrenal insufficiency may occur in those who do not have Addison's disease, such as those who have received cortisone for various reasons, usually a minimum of 20 mg daily for at least 5 days. *Symptoms* include:

- fever
- nausea and vomiting, abdominal pain
- weakness and general fatigue
- disorientation, confusion
- hypotensive shock
- dehydration
- electrolyte imbalance with hyperkalemia, hypercalcemia, hypoglycemia and hyponatremia.

Immediate *treatment* includes:

- IV fluids in large volume
- glucocorticoid
- dextrose 50% if indicated (hypoglycemia)
- mineralocorticoid may be needed after IV solutions.
- The precipitating cause must be identified and treated as well.

Cushing Syndrome

Cushing syndrome is caused by increased production of cortisol from a variety of etiologies:

- excess of adrenocorticotropic hormone (ACTH) causing adrenal hyperplasia; hypersecretion of glucocorticoids usually related to neoplasms; extrapituitary neoplasms causing autonomous secretion of ACTH; Iatrogenic, resulting from exogenous corticosteroids
- treatment with corticosteroids

Symptoms include:

- changes in fat distribution with truncal obesity, supraclavicular fat pads, and fat pads on back of neck, moon face, large abdomen, weight gain; increased bruising and poor wound healing
- Hypertension; hypokalemia; hyperglycemia
- virilization with increased hirsutism and acne
- kyphosis with depressed linear growth.

Treatment depends upon the cause. If caused by medications, such as prednisone, slow withdrawal of the medication should reverse symptoms over time. Giving medications in early morning on alternate days may reduce symptoms. In some cases, bilateral adrenalectomy and replacement hormone therapy (as for Addison's disease) is indicated.

Diabetes Insipidus

Diabetes insipidus (DI) **is** caused by a deficiency of the antidiuretic hormone (ADH), or vasopressin. DI may develop secondary to head trauma, primary brain tumor, meningitis, encephalitis, surgical ablation or irradiation of the pituitary gland, or metastatic tumors. This is different from congenital nephrogenic diabetes insipidus, in which production of ADH is normal but the renal tubules do not respond; however, the symptoms are the same. *Symptoms* include:

- polydipsia
- polyuria
- Patients may exhibit excessive thirst and may drink excessively, 2 to 20 liters a day, without relief of thirst. Withholding fluids results in dehydration but polyuria continues.

Treatment includes:

- Vasopressin tannate is available as an injection (IM or subcutaneous) or nasal spray. Injectable forms may last up to 72 hours.
- Desmopressin acetate is available as a nasal spray or oral medication and is usually taken twice daily. Water intoxication can occur with overdose.

SIADH

Syndrome of inappropriate secretion of antidiuretic hormone (SIADH) is related to hypersecretion of the posterior pituitary gland. This causes the kidneys to reabsorb fluids, resulting in fluid retention, and triggers a decrease in sodium levels (dilutional hyponatremia), resulting in production of only concentrated urine. This syndrome may result from CNS disorders, such as brain trauma, surgery, or tumors. It may also be triggered by other disorders, such as tumors of various organs, pneumothorax, acute pneumonia, and other lung disorders. Some medications (vincristine, phenothiazines, tricyclic antidepressants, and thiazide diuretics) may also trigger SIADH. *Symptoms* include:

- anorexia with nausea and vomiting
- irritability
- stomach cramps

- alterations of personality
- increasing neurological dysfunction, including stupor and seizures, related to progressive sodium depletion.

Treatment includes identifying and treating underlying cause, fluid restriction, and loop diuretics (furosemide).

Hematology

Lab Tests

A number of different tests are used to evaluate the condition and production of RBCs in addition to the RBC count:

- Hemoglobin: Carries oxygen and is decreased in anemia and increased in polycythemia. Normal values:
    - Men older than18 years: 14 to 17.46 g/dL
    - Women older than18 years: 12 to 16 g/dL
- Hematocrit: Indicates the proportion of RBCs in a liter of blood (usually about 3 times the hemoglobin number). Normal values:
    - Men older than18 years: 45% to 52%.
    - Women older than18 years: 36% to 48%
- Mean corpuscular volume (MCV): Indicates the size of RBCs and can differentiate types of anemia. For adults, less than 80 is microcytic and greater than 100 is macrocytic. Normal values:
    - Men older than 18 years: 84 to 96 mcm^3
    - Women older than18 years: 76 to 96 mcm^3
- Reticulocyte count: measures marrow production and should rise with anemia. Normal values:
    - 0.5% to 1.5% of total RBCs.

Anemias

Red blood cells (RBCs or erythrocytes) are biconcave disks that contain hemoglobin (95% of mass), which carries oxygen throughout the body. The heme portion of the cell contains iron, which binds to the oxygen. RBCs live about 120 days after which they are destroyed and their hemoglobin is recycled or excreted. Normal values of RBC count vary by gender:

- Men older than 18 years: 4.5 to 5.5 million per mm^3
- Women older than18 years: 4 to 5 million per mm^3

The most common disorders of RBCs are those that interfere with production, leading to various types of anemia:

- blood loss
- hemolysis
- bone marrow failure.

The morphology of RBCs may vary depending upon the type of anemia:

- Size: normocytes, microcytes, macrocytes
- Shape: spherocytes (round), poikilocytes (irregular), drepanocytes (sickled)
- Color (reflecting concentration of hemoglobin): normochromic, hypochromic.

Anemia results in a decrease in oxygen transportation and decreased perfusion throughout the body, causing the heart to compensate by increasing cardiac output. As the blood becomes less viscous, there is decreased peripheral resistance, so more blood is pumped to the heart, and this increased flow can cause turbulence that results in a heart murmur and, if severe or prolonged, heart failure. Anemia is commonly caused by hemorrhage, hemolysis, hematopoiesis, or dietary iron deficiency in women who are menstruating. *Symptoms* include:

- general malaise and weakness
- poor feeding/ anorexia
- pallor
- shortness of breath on exertion
- headache, dizziness
- apathy, depression, decreased attention span, slowed thought processes
- shock symptoms (with severe blood loss): tachycardia, hypotension, poor peripheral circulation, and pallor.

Treatment:

- Identification and treatment of underlying cause.
- Blood or blood components as indicated.
- Supportive care: oxygen, IV fluids.
- Splenectomy (for hemolytic anemias).

Anemia results in a decrease in oxygen transportation and decreased perfusion throughout the body, causing the heart to compensate by increasing cardiac output. As the blood becomes less viscous, there is decreased peripheral resistance, so more blood is pumped to the heart, and this increased flow can cause turbulence that results in a heart murmur and, if severe or prolonged, heart failure. Anemia is commonly caused by hemorrhage, hemolysis, hematopoiesis, or dietary iron deficiency in women who are menstruating. Children can tolerate low oxygen levels better than adults; however, growth and sexual development may be delayed with chronic anemia. *Symptoms* include:

- general malaise and weakness, poor feeding/ anorexia
- pallor, shortness of breath on exertion
- headache, dizziness, apathy, depression, decreased attention span, slowed thought processes
- shock symptoms (with severe blood loss): tachycardia, hypotension, poor peripheral circulation, and pallor.

Treatment:

- Treatment of underlying cause.
- Blood or blood components as indicated.
- Supportive care: oxygen, IV fluids.
- Referral for splenectomy (hemolytic anemias).

COAGULOPATHIES

IDIOPATHIC THROMBOCYTOPENIA PURPURA

Idiopathic thrombocytopenia purpura is an autoimmune condition in which the thrombocyte (platelet) count is below normal (less than 150,000/mm^3) but the other blood values are normal, resulting in purple bruises and petechiae on the skin and mucous membranes from superficial bleeding. The acute form (lasting less than 6 months) occurs primarily in children after viral infections or live virus vaccination. The chronic form (lasting longer than 6 months) is more common in adults (primarily women) but can occur at any age, and the cause is unknown. Other *symptoms* include menorrhagia, epistaxis, gastrointestinal (GI) bleeding, and bleeding gums.

Retinal and cerebral hemorrhage (rare) may occur. Diagnosis includes: CBC and platelet count. *Treatment* includes:

- corticosteroids to increase platelet count
- IV immune globulin for severe bleeding, platelet count less than 50,000 (adults), or (pediatrics) platelet count less than 20,000
- hemorrhage: volume replacement if indicated as for hypovolemic shock
- phase 2 studies of eltrombopag (50 and 75 mg daily) have been complete, showing the drug effective in increasing platelet count within 1 week.

Polycythemia Vera

Polycythemia is a condition in which there is abnormal production of blood cells in the bone marrow. Erythrocytes (red blood cells) are primarily affected. The disease is more common in men older than 40 years of age. Polycythemia may be primary or secondary, related to conditions causing hypoxia. The blood increases in viscosity, resulting in a number of *symptoms*:

- dizziness, headache, weakness, and fatigue
- dyspnea, especially when supine.
- flushing of skin, skin discoloration (blue-tinged), red lesions
- Itching after warm bath
- left upper abdominal fullness and splenomegaly
- phlebitis from blood clots
- vision disturbances.

Complications include stroke, hemorrhage, and heart failure. *Diagnosis* includes CBC with differential, chemistry panel, bone marrow biopsy, Vitamin B12 level, and red cell mass greater than 25% above normal. *Treatment* includes:

- phlebotomy to remove 500 mL (lesser amounts for children) of blood to decrease blood viscosity, repeated weekly until hematocrit stable (less than 45)
- referral for chemotherapy to suppress marrow production: hydroxyurea
- interferon to decrease need for phlebotomy

DIC

Disseminated intravascular coagulation (DIC) (consumption coagulopathy) is a secondary disorder that is triggered by another, such as trauma, congenital heart disease, necrotizing enterocolitis, sepsis, and severe viral infections. DIC triggers both coagulation and hemorrhage through a complex series of events that includes trauma that causes tissue factor (transmembrane glycoprotein) to enter the circulation and bind with coagulation factors, triggering the coagulation cascade. This stimulates thrombin to convert fibrinogen to fibrin, causing aggregation and destruction of platelets and forming clots that can be disseminated throughout the intravascular system. These clots increase in size as platelets adhere to the clots, causing blockage of both the microvascular systems and larger vessels, and this can result in ischemia and necrosis. Clot formation triggers fibrinolysis and plasmin to breakdown fibrin and fibrinogen, causing destruction of clotting factors, resulting in hemorrhage. Both processes, clotting and hemorrhage, continue at the same time, placing the patient at high risk for death, even with treatment.

The onset of disseminated intravascular coagulation (DIC) symptoms may be very rapid or a slower chronic progression from a disease, such as in children with large vascular malformations. *Symptoms* include:

- bleeding from surgical or venous puncture sites
- bleeding from umbilicus and trachea in newborns
- evidence of GI bleeding with distention, bloody diarrhea

- hypotension and acute symptoms of shock
- petechiae and purpura with extensive bleeding into the tissues
- laboratory abnormalities:
    - prolonged prothrombin and partial prothrombin times.
    - decreased platelet counts and fragmented RBCs.
    - decreased fibrinogen.

Those who develop the chronic manifestation of the disease usually have fewer acute symptoms and may slowly develop ecchymosis or bleeding wounds. *Treatment* varies and includes:

- identifying and treating underlying cause
- replacement blood products, such as platelets and fresh frozen plasma
- anticoagulation therapy (heparin) to increase clotting time
- cryoprecipitate to increase fibrinogen levels
- coagulation inhibitors and coagulation factors

HEMOPHILIA

Hemophilia is an inherited disorder in which the person lacks adequate clotting factors. There are 3 types:

- Type A: lack of clotting factor VIII (90% of cases)
- Type B: lack of clotting factor IX
- Type C: lack of clotting factor XI (affects both sexes, rarely occurs in the United States).

Both Type A and B are usually X-linked disorders, affecting only males. The severity of the disease depends on the amount of clotting factor in the blood. *Symptoms* include:

- bleeding with severe trauma or stress (mild cases)
- unexplained bruises, bleeding, swelling, joint pain
- spontaneous hemorrhage (severe cases), often in the joints but can be anywhere in the body
- epistaxis.

First symptoms often occur during infancy when the child becomes active, resulting in frequent bruises. *Treatment* includes:

- desmopressin parenterally or nasally to stimulate production of clotting factor (mild cases)
- infusions of clotting factor from donated blood or recombinant clotting factors (genetically engineered)
- infusions of plasma (type C)

HITTS

Heparin-induced thrombocytopenia and thrombosis syndrome (HITTS) occurs in patients receiving heparin for anticoagulation. There are 2 types:

- *Type I* is a transient condition occurring within a few days and causing depletion of platelets (less than 100,000 mm^3), but heparin may be continued as the condition usually resolves without intervention.

- *Type II* is an autoimmune reaction to heparin that occurs in 3% to 5% of those receiving unfractionated heparin and also occurs with low molecular weight heparin. It is characterized by low platelets (less than 50,000 mm^3) that are at least 50% below baseline. Onset is 5 to 14 days but can occur within hours of reheparinization. Death rates are 30% or less. Heparin-antibody complexes form and release platelet factor 4 (PF4), which attracts heparin molecules and adheres to platelets and endothelial lining, stimulating thrombin and platelet clumping. This puts the patient at risk for thrombosis and vessel occlusion rather than hemorrhage, causing stroke, myocardial infarction, and limb ischemia with symptoms associated with the site of thrombosis. *Treatment* includes:
    - discontinuation of heparin
    - direct thrombin inhibitors (lepirudin, argatroban).

Immune Disorders

Antiretroviral Agents

There are 4 primary classes of antiretroviral agents used for the treatment of HIV/AIDS:

- *Non-nucleoside reverse transcriptase inhibitors* (NNRTIs), such as delavirdine (Rescriptor®), efavirenz (Sustiva®), and nevirapine (Viramune®), bind to reverse transcriptase and disable it. Reverse transcriptase is a protein required for HIV replication.
- *Nucleoside reverse transcriptase inhibitors* (NRTIs), such as abacavir (Ziagen®), abacavir (Epzicom®), zidovudine (AZT®), and lamivudine (Epivir®), are defective versions of building blocks necessary for replication. When HIV binds to the defective version, it is unable to complete replication.
- *Protease inhibitors* (PIs) disable the protein protease, which HIV requires in order to replicate. PIs include amprenavir (Agenerase®), indinavir (Crixivan®), and nelfinavir (Viracept®).
- *Fusion inhibitors* such as enfuvirtide (Fuzeon®) are entry blockers.

Immunosuppression

Immunosuppression, whether because of diseases such as AIDS or drugs used for organ transplantation, increases the risk of the development of neoplasms.

- *Heart transplantations*: There is about a 6% risk of developing a solid tumor after transplantation. The most common types are skin (basal cell, squamous cell, Meckel cell carcinoma, and melanoma) and lung cancers, although a variety of cancers, including liver, breast, uterine, testicular, and bladder, have been reported.
- *All transplantations*: The most common tumors associated with all types of transplantations are skin cancers, lymphomas, cervical cancer, and liver cancer.
- *AIDS*: There has been a substantial decline in the rate of Kaposi sarcoma and non-Hodgkin lymphoma with improvement in treatment of AIDS; however, risk of cervical cancer remains high, and there has been an increased incidence of Hodgkin lymphoma.

Studies have indicated that pretreating transplantation patients with immunosuppressant antithymocyte globulin and decreasing postoperative immunosuppression may reduce the risk of cancer.

HIV

Human immunodeficiency virus (HIV) is a slow-acting retrovirus of the genus lentivirus. HIV binds with cells that have CD4 receptors, primarily CD4+ T cells and other cells of the immune system, enters the cells, and begins replicating. Host cells are destroyed in a number of ways:

- Disruption of cell wall or cellular function may be caused after large numbers of replicated viral cells bud through the cell membrane or build up inside the cell.
- Formation of syncytia occurs when cells infected with HIV fuse with nearby cells creating giant cells, thus allowing HIV to spread from one cell to many.

- Apoptosis, or cell death, occurs when HIV sends a signal to uninfected cells, causing them to self-destruct.
- Binding to cell surface of uninfected cell by HIV gives the appearance that the cell is infected, causing it to be targeted by killer T cells as part of the immune response.

HIV is spread through blood or other bodily fluids and blood-contaminated equipment.

AIDS

Acquired immunodeficiency syndrome (AIDS) is a progression of infection with human immunodeficiency virus (HIV). AIDS is diagnosed when the following criteria are met: HIV infection; CD4 count less than 200 cells/mm^3

AIDS-defining condition, such as opportunistic infections (cytomegalovirus, tuberculosis), wasting syndrome, neoplasms (Kaposi sarcoma), or AIDS dementia complex.

Because there is such a wide range of AIDS-defining conditions, the patient may present with many types of *symptoms*, depending upon the diagnosis, but more than half of AIDS patients exhibit: Fever, lymphadenopathy, pharyngitis, rash, myalgia/arthralgia. It is important to review the following: CD4 counts, to determine immune status, WBC and differential for signs of infection, cultures to help identify any infective agents, complete blood cell count to evaluate for signs of bleeding or thrombocytopenia.

Treatment aims to cure or manage opportunistic conditions and control underlying HIV infection through highly active antiretroviral therapy (HAART), 3 or more drugs used concurrently.

Rheumatoid Arthritis

The autoimmune reaction of rheumatoid arthritis primarily affects the synovial tissue. Essentially, phagocytosis (neutrophils) produce enzymes (such as proteinase) in the joints that break down the collagen, cause proliferation of the synovial membrane and pannus formation that destroys cartilage and bone. It begins with antigen presentation to T cells and subsequent proliferation of both B and T cells, causing angiogenesis in the synovial lining of the joints, resulting in swelling, pain, and stiffness. Neutrophils begin to accumulate in the synovial fluid and cells proliferate, but in the initial stages there is no invasion of the cartilage; however, swelling and effusions increase with possible development of nodules. This progresses to synovitis with early pannus (inflammatory synovial tissue) invasion and chondrocyte activation. Proteinase begins to cause degradation of the cartilage as symptoms worsen. Finally, there is erosion of the subchondral bone and pannus invasion of the cartilage with proliferation of chondrocytes and weakening of ligaments, causing joint instability, contractures, and increasing systemic manifestations.

Osteoarthritis and Rheumatoid Arthritis

There are many different types of arthritis, but the 2 most common are osteoarthritis and rheumatoid arthritis. There are distinctive differences:

Osteoarthritis	Rheumatoid arthritis
Idiopathic or previous injury	Systemic autoimmune inflammatory disorder (etiology unknown)
Slowly progressive with symptoms > 60 years of age	Acute onset beginning in hands, wrists, feet at 25 to 50 years of age
Cartilage deterioration	Joint inflammation and deformity
Pain increases with use/weightbearing. Stiffness develops	Pain, stiffness, swelling, erythema, nodules, and lack of function in affected joints, and generalized weakness, fatigue, weight loss, and fever
Local and unilateral	Systemic and bilateral and symmetric

Osteoarthritis	Rheumatoid arthritis
NSAIDs, heat, weight reduction, joint rest, orthotic devices, postural exercises	Light exercise to prevent contractures. Medications: Salicylates (ASA), NSAIDs, COX-2 inhibitors (Celebrex®)

Gout

Gout (metabolic arthritis) is a group of conditions associated with a defect of purine metabolism that results in hyperuricemia with oversecretion of uric acid, decreased excretion of uric acid, or a combination. The increased uric acid levels can cause monosodium urate crystal depositions in the joints, resulting in severe articular and periarticular inflammation. With chronic gout, sodium urate crystals, called tophi, accumulate in peripheral body areas, such as the great toe (75%), hands, and ears, although other joints may be affected as well. *Symptoms* include abrupt onset of pain with erythema and edema lasting 3 to 10 days. Attacks become more frequent over time and some may develop kidney stones. Diagnosis is based on clinical examination, history, and uric acid level higher than 7 mg/dL. *Treatment* includes:

- restriction of high-purine foods (organ meats) and alcohol
- weight-control methods
- Acute medications:
  - NSAIDs
  - colchicine
- Prophylactic medications for chronic episodes:
  - probenecid (to prevent tophi formation)
  - allopurinol (to prevent formation of uric acid).

Fibromyalgia

Fibromyalgia is a complex syndrome of disorders that include fatigue, chronic generalized muscle pain, and focal areas of tenderness persisting for at least 3 months. The cause of fibromyalgia is not clear and has only recently been recognized as a distinct disorder. Symptoms vary widely but can include:

- pain and stiffness unresponsive to treatment, persisting for months
- sleep disorders
- irritable bowel syndrome
- stiffness in neck and shoulders associated with headache and pain in face
- sensitivity to odor, noises, and lights
- mood disorders, such as depression or anxiety
- dysmenorrhea
- paresthesia in hands and feet.

Diagnosis is by clinical exam and ruling out other disorders. *Treatment* includes:

- Analgesia: acetaminophen, tramadol, or NSAIDs
- Antidepressants such as amitriptyline, nortriptyline, or fluoxetine. Duloxetine and venlafaxine have been shown to reduce pain.
- Pregabalin is the first FDA-approved treatment for the pain of fibromyalgia.
- Referral for physical therapy and/or cognitive therapy

Lupus Erythematosus

Systemic lupus erythematosus is a systemic reaction to collagen or connective tissue in the body, believed triggered by an antibody-antigen immune response to an environmental agent, resulting in widespread damage of vessels and organs, primarily in females. Onset is usually at 9 to 15 years of age and is more common in African American, Hispanic, and Asian girls than Caucasian. *Symptoms* vary widely and may include:

- "butterfly" rash (scaly erythematous maculopapular patches) on face, chest, and arms
- arthritic-type pain, stiffness, and swelling of joints
- CNS involvement with seizures, headache, and psychosis
- heart (pericarditis) and lung (pleurisy) inflammation
- kidney failure
- anemia (erythrocytopenia)
- spleen, liver, and lymph nodes enlarged
- GI symptoms: nausea, vomiting, pain, and hepatitis.

Treatment varies according to severity of disease and includes:

- NSAIDs for pain and inflammation
- steroids for organ inflammation
- antimalarial drugs for skin involvement
- immunosuppressant agents if steroids not adequate

Organ Transplantation

HSCT

Hematopoietic stem cell transplantation (HSCT) from stem cells harvested from bone marrow, peripheral blood, or cord blood may be done for leukemia, some solid tumors, aplastic anemia, genetic, or immune deficiency disorders. HCST offers long-term remission, but the risks are high. Graft-versus-host disease (GVHD) is a common complication.

- Allogenic transplants use donor stem cells from family members or an unrelated donor.
- Syngenic transplants are from identical twins.
- Autologous transplants, using the patient's stem cells, have a lower risk than allogenic transplants, but if used for leukemia, cancer cells may inadvertently be transplanted with the cells.

Transplants from related donors have lower rates of GVHD and lower mortality rates. Transplantation is done through IV transfusion. If used for cancers that affect the bone marrow, such as leukemia, the patient must undergo either ablative doses of chemotherapy or total body irradiation to destroy the bone marrow and disease that exists prior to transplantation, which leaves the patient susceptible to infection and disease.

Liver Transplantations

Liver transplantation is often the only effective treatment for end-stage liver disease or abnormalities (extrahepatic biliary atresia), metabolic diseases (Wilson disease), toxic necrosis (viral infections, drugs), cirrhosis, and malignancies. Liver transplants are obtained from both cadaveric and living donors because the liver can regenerate. The right lobe is divided into anterior and posterior segments and the left into lateral and medial segments. One cadaver liver can be divided for more than one transplantation. In adult living donors, either an entire lobe or one segment, such as the left lateral lobe, is removed; this size is adequate for small children, who often receive transplants in the first 2 years. The blood type of donors must be compatible with the recipient's. Patients receive the donor organ and begin immunosuppressive drugs to prevent rejection of the organ, with risk for rejection the greatest in the first 3 months.

Heart Transplantations

Heart transplantation is similar to other open-heart procedures in that cardiopulmonary bypass is needed during the procedure. The sternotomy and thymectomy is performed and then the pericardial sac is opened to expose the heart. If the donor heart is larger than the recipient's, the left pericardium, sparing the phrenic nerve, may be removed. The orthotopic procedure is the most commonly used. In this procedure, the posterior portion of the left atrium is left for attachment of the new heart but the rest of the heart is excised. The donor heart may be trimmed and is sutured to fit with the remnants of the old heart. Once the new heart is in place, the heart is taken off bypass and is stimulated to begin contractions. In heterotopic transplantation (rare), the new heart is sutured to the old heart, joining the chambers to create a "double" heart.

POSTOPERATIVE MANAGEMENT

Postoperative management of heart transplant patients is similar to that of other cardiac surgeries. Treatments include:

- *Mechanical ventilation* is used initially, but respiratory care with adequate ventilation must be monitored constantly, especially if the donor heart was larger than the native heart, resulting in compression of the lungs.
- *IV fluids* and various medications, such as sedation and vasodilators, will be administered.
- *Prostaglandin* is continued for 1 to 2 days if used preoperatively to preclude rebound pulmonary hypertension.
- *Immunosuppression therapy,* such as antithymocyte globulin, azathioprine, cyclosporine, or tacrolimus (Prograf®), may be used for immunosuppression, as well as corticosteroids (methylprednisolone). IV immunosuppressive drugs are given after surgery but these are switched to oral medications when possible. Protocols are established at each institution and may vary. Medication doses are age-dependent.

The risk for rejection is the greatest in the first few month and close follow-up with regular routine laboratory tests, including echocardiograms, chest x-rays, and blood tests, must be done.

LUNG TRANSPLANTATION

Lung transplantation is the replacement of one or both lungs, and sometimes a lobe, with donor organs. Combined heart and lung transplants are much less common now than in earlier surgeries. Lung transplantation is often indicated because of damage to the lungs from COPD. Conditions requiring transplantation include:

- emphysema resulting in shunting and ineffective ventilation
- cystic fibrosis resulting in recurrent infections, pneumonia, and mucus production that clogs airways and interferes with ventilation
- pulmonary fibrosis creating excessive scarring in lung tissue
- pulmonary hypertension preventing adequate blood flow to the lungs.

Criteria for recipients include:

- end-stage pulmonary disease nonresponsive to treatment
- lack of significant medical disease that may interfere with progress
- condition substantially limits activities
- life expectancy is limited by condition
- potential for rehabilitation exists
- nutritional status is adequate to promote and support healing
- support system and psychosocial profile are adequate.

Risk Factors

Heart and/or lung transplant patients are especially susceptible to bacterial pulmonary infections, with infections occurring in 35% to 48% of hosts. Some risk factors place patients at increased risk:

- Cytomegalovirus (CMV)–positive donor places seronegative heart and/or lung transplant patients at increased risk for postoperative CMV pneumonia, invasive aspergillosis, and pulmonary bacterial infections.
- Preoperative colonization of Aspergillus fumigatus in cystic fibrosis patients poses the risk of postoperative tracheobronchial aspergillosis.
- Colonization of resistant Pseudomonas strains in the damaged lungs, especially in cystic fibrosis patients, can result in residual infection in other parts of the respiratory tract, providing a source of infection for the donor organs.
- Invasive devices such as central venous lines, circulatory assist devices, and ventilators may result in colonization and infection, especially pneumonia and sternal surgical-site infections.
- Decreased ability to cough and clear mucous because of loss of cough reflex, pain, or weakness can contribute to pneumonia.

Kidney Transplantation

Kidney transplantation is indicated for a wide range of disorders, including kidney disease requiring dialysis, congenital abnormalities with urinary blockage, glomerulonephritis, and hemolytic uremic syndrome. Diabetes is the primary cause of kidney disease requiring transplantation. Adult cadaveric or living donor organs may be used. Usually the diseased kidney is not removed, so the donor kidney is placed in a different position, usually the iliac fossa. Steroids, such as prednisone, have been used with tacrolimus for immunosuppression, but recent studies indicate that extended use of daclizumab can provide equally effective steroid-free immunosuppression, with fewer side effects. Other studies show that preconditioning with alemtuzumab and tacrolimus allows avoidance of steroids. However, some immunosuppressive drugs must be taken throughout life to prevent rejection. Acute rejection can occur during the first 60 days, but the danger of rejection may be long-term. Kidney transplants usually last 10 to 15 years before another transplant or dialysis is needed.

Pancreas Transplantation

Pancreas transplantation is done to treat type 1 (insulin-dependent) diabetes mellitus. Because of the danger of rejection and the need for immunosuppressive drugs, transplantation is usually done for those with severe symptoms. Pancreas organs are obtained from cadaveric or living donors who have surgical removal of half of their pancreas. Most pancreas transplantations (85%) are done in conjunction with kidney transplantations or following kidney transplantations (10%) because of kidney damage caused by diabetes. Many patients are receiving dialysis prior to surgery. Another procedure that is still fairly new is islet transplantation, which involves isolating islet cells from a donor organ and then transplanting them by infusion into the portal vein of the liver. Patients often require 2 or 3 transplants, but some achieve insulin independence. This procedure is still considered experimental but shows promise. Both pancreas and islet cell transplantations require immunosuppression.

Graft-Versus-Host Disease

GVHD is an immunological response to "foreign" tissue (such as a transplanted organ or nonirradiated blood transfusion). GVHD is one of the major causes of morbidity and mortality after transplantations, so immunosuppression is provided before, during, and after transplantations (usually about 6 months for allogenic stem cell transplantation and lifelong for solid organs). GVHD may be acute (fewer than 100 days after transplantation) or chronic (more than 100 days after transplantation). *Symptoms* may involve many organs, such as the skin, the GI tract, and the liver. Patients may experience diffuse, lacy maculopapular rash, nausea, vomiting, diarrhea, sloughing of mucosal tissue, and increasing bilirubin. GVHD is staged according to severity of symptoms related to the skin, GI system, and liver, with each system graded 1 to 4, depending upon severity. *Treatment* includes corticosteroids to suppress the immune response.

SICKLE CELL CRISIS

SICKLE CELL DISEASE

Sickle cell disease is a recessive genetic disorder of chromosome 11, causing hemoglobin to be defective so that red blood cells (RBCs) are sickle-shaped and inflexible, resulting in their accumulating in small vessels and causing painful blockage. While normal RBCs survive 120 days, sickled cells may survive only 10 to 20 days, stressing the bone marrow that cannot produce fast enough and resulting in severe anemia. There are 5 variations of sickle cell disease, with sickle cell anemia the most severe. Different types of crises occur (aplastic, hemolytic, vaso-occlusive, and sequestrating), which cause infarctions in organs, severe pain, damage to organs, and rapid enlargement of liver and spleen Complications include anemia, acute chest syndrome, congestive heart failure, strokes, delayed growth, infections, pulmonary hypertension, liver and kidney disorders, retinopathy, seizures, and osteonecrosis. Sickle cell disease occurs almost exclusively in African Americans in the United States, with 8% to 10% carriers.

Review Video: Sickle Cell Disease
Visit mometrix.com/academy and enter code: 603869

SICKLE CELL DISEASE AND CRISIS

Sickle cell disease and crisis *treatment* includes:

- IV fluids to prevent dehydration.
- Analgesics (morphine) during painful crises.
- Folic acid for anemia.
- Oxygen for congestive heart failure or pulmonary disease.
- Blood transfusions with chelation therapy to remove excess iron OR erythropheresis, in which red cells are removed and replaced with healthy cells, either autologous or from a donor.
- HSCT is the only curative treatment, but immunosuppressive drugs must be used and success rates are only about 85%, so the procedure is only used on those at high risk. It requires ablation of bone marrow, placing the patient at increased risk.
- Partial chimerism uses a mixture of the donor and the recipient's bone marrow stem cells, and does not require ablation of bone marrow. It is showing good success.

Neurology

CEREBROVASCULAR DISORDERS

CEREBRAL ANEURYSMS

Cerebral aneurysms, weakening and dilation of a cerebral artery, are usually congenital (90%) while the remaining (10%) result from direct trauma or infection. Aneurysms usually range from 2 to 7 mm and occur in the circle of Willis at the base of the brain. A rupturing aneurysm may decrease perfusion as well as increase pressure on surrounding brain tissue. Cerebral aneurysms are classified as follows:

- *Berry/saccular:* The most common congenital type occurs at a bifurcation and grows from the base on a stem, usually at the circle of Willis.
- *Fusiform:* Large (greater than 2.5 cm) and irregular and rarely ruptures but causes increased intracranial pressure. Usually involves the internal carotid or vertebrobasilar artery.
- *Mycotic:* Rare type that occurs secondary to bacterial infection and a septic emboli.
- *Dissecting:* Wall is torn apart and blood enters layers. This may occur during angiography or secondary to trauma or disease.
- *Traumatic Charcot-Bouchard (pseudoaneurysm):* Small lesion resulting from chronic hypertension.

Arteriovenous Malformation

Arteriovenous malformation (AVM) is a congenital abnormality of a tangle of dilated arteries and veins without a capillary bed. AVMs can occur anywhere in the brain and may cause no significant problems. Usually the AVM is "fed" by one or more cerebral arteries, which enlarge over time, shunting more blood through the AVM. The veins also enlarge in response to increased arterial blood flow because of the lack of a capillary bridge between the two. Because vein walls are thinner and lack the muscle layer of an artery, the veins tend to rupture as the AVM becomes larger, causing a subarachnoid hemorrhage. Chronic ischemia that may be related to the AVM can result in cerebral atrophy. Sometimes small leaks usually accompanied by headache and nausea and vomiting may occur before rupture. AVMs may cause a wide range of neurological *symptoms*, including changes in mentation, dizziness, sensory abnormalities, confusion, and dementia. *Treatment* includes:

- supportive management of symptoms
- surgical repair or focused irradiation (definitive treatments).

Ischemic Stroke

Strokes (brain attacks, cerebrovascular accidents) result when there is interruption of the blood flow to an area of the brain. The two basic types are ischemic and hemorrhagic. About 80% are ischemic, resulting from blockage of an artery supplying the brain:

- *Thrombosis* in a large artery, usually resulting from atherosclerosis, may block circulation to a large area of the brain. It is most common in elderly persons and may occur suddenly or after episodes of transient ischemic attacks.
- *Lacunar infarct* (penetrating thrombosis in small artery) is most common in those with diabetes mellitus and/or hypertension.
- *Embolism* travels through the arterial system and lodges in the brain, most commonly in the left middle cerebral artery. An embolism may be cardiogenic, resulting from cardiac arrhythmia or surgery. An embolism usually occurs rapidly with no warning signs.
- *Cryptogenic* has no identifiable cause

Hemorrhagic Stroke

Hemorrhagic strokes account for about 20% of all people admitted to the hospital for strokes. They result from a ruptured cerebral artery, causing not only lack of oxygen and nutrients but also edema that causes widespread pressure and damage:

- *Intracerebral* is bleeding into the substance of the brain from an artery in the central lobes, basal ganglia, pons, or cerebellum. Intracerebral hemorrhage usually results from atherosclerotic degenerative changes, hypertension, brain tumors, anticoagulation therapy, or some illicit drugs, such as crack and cocaine. Onset is often sudden and may cause death.
- *Intracranial aneurysm* occurs with ballooning cerebral artery ruptures, most commonly at the circle of Willis.
- *AVM* is a tangle of dilated arteries and veins without a capillary bed. This is a congenital abnormality. Rupture of AVMs is a cause of brain attack in younger adults.
- *Subarachnoid hemorrhage* is bleeding in the space between the meninges and brain, resulting from aneurysm, AVM, or trauma. This type of hemorrhage compresses brain tissue.

Stroke Symptoms

Strokes most commonly occur in the right or left hemisphere, but the exact location and the extent of brain damage affects the type of presenting symptoms. If the frontal area of either side is involved, there tends to be memory and learning deficits. Some symptoms are common to specific areas and help to identify the area involved:

Right hemisphere: This results in left paralysis or paresis and a left visual field deficit that may cause spatial and perceptual disturbances so that people may have difficulty judging distance. Fine motor skills may be impacted, resulting in trouble dressing or handling tools. People may become impulsive and exhibit poor judgment, often denying impairment. Left-sided neglect (lack of perception of things on the left side) may occur. Difficulty following directions, short-term memory loss, and depression are also common. Language skills usually remain intact.

Symptoms of strokes vary according to the area of the brain affected:

- *Left hemisphere*: This results in right paralysis or paresis and a right visual field defect. Depression is common and people often exhibit slow, cautious behavior, requiring repeated instruction and reinforcement for simple tasks. Short-term memory loss and difficulty learning new material or understanding generalizations are common. Difficulty with mathematics, reading, writing, and reasoning may occur. Aphasia (expressive, receptive, or global) is common.
- *Brain stem:* Because the brain stem controls respiration and cardiac function, a brain attack frequently causes death, but those who survive may have a number of problems, including respiratory and cardiac abnormalities. Strokes may involve motor or sensory impairment or both.
- *Cerebellum:* This area controls balance and coordination. Strokes in the cerebellum are rare but may result in ataxia, nausea, and vomiting, and headaches and dizziness or vertigo.

Medical Management

Medical management of ischemic strokes with tissue plasminogen activator (tPA), the primary treatment, should be initiated within 3 hours:

- *Thrombolytic medication* (tPA) is produced by recombinant DNA and is used to dissolve fibrin clots. It is given intravenously (0.9mg/kg up to 90 mg) with 10% injected as an initial bolus and the rest over the next hour.
- *Antihypertensives* if mean arterial pressure (MAP) greater than 130 mm HG or systolic BP greater than 220 mm Hg.
- *Cooling* to reduce hyperthermia. *Osmotic diuretics* (mannitol), hypertonic saline, loop diuretics (furosemide), and/or corticosteroids (dexamethasone) to decrease cerebral edema and intracranial pressure. *Aspirin/Anticoagulation* may be used with embolism.
- *Stool softeners* to prevent constipation.

Monitor and treat hyperglycemia.

- Contraindications to thrombolytic therapy include:
- evidence of cerebral or subarachnoid hemorrhage or other internal bleeding; recent stroke, head trauma, or surgery
- history of intracranial hemorrhage; uncontrolled hypertension
- Seizures; intracranial AVM, neoplasm, or aneurysm
- current anticoagulation therapy; low platelet count (less than $100{,}000/mm^3$).

Disorders of the Spine

Lumbosacral Pain

Lumbosacral (low back) pain may be related to strain, muscular weakness, osteoarthritis, spinal stenosis, herniated disks, vertebral fractures, bony metastasis, infection, or other musculoskeletal disorders. Disk herniation or other joint changes put pressure on nerves leaving the spinal cord, causing pain to radiate along the nerve. Pain may be acute or chronic (greater than 3 months). *Symptoms* include: local or pain radiating down the leg (radiculopathy), impaired gait and reflexes, difference in leg lengths, decreased motor strength, and alteration of sensation, including numbness. *Diagnosis* is by careful clinical examination and history as well as x-ray (fractures, scoliosis, dislocations), CT (identifies underlying problems), magnetic resonance imaging (MRI) (spinal pathology), and/or electromyography (EMG) and nerve conduction studies. Diagnostic studies may be deferred in many cases for 4 to 6 weeks as symptoms may resolve over time. *Treatments* for nonspecific back pain include:

- Analgesia: acetaminophen, NSAIDs, opiates.
- Encourage activity to tolerance but not bed rest.
- Muscle relaxants: diazepam 5 to 10 mg every 6 to 8 hours.
- Cold compresses and/or heart compresses.

Disorders of the Spine

There are a number of spinal disorders that may require surgical repair, such as spinal fusion:

- *Kyphosis*, a convex angulation of the thoracic spine, may be secondary to conditions such as arthritis or compression fractures, or may be postural, resulting from skeletal growth faster than muscular. Exercises may help postural kyphosis.
- *Lordosis,* an often painful concave angulation of the lumbar spine, frequently associated with obesity, flexion hip contracture, and slipped femoral capital epiphysis. Exercises may give some relief but not a permanent cure.
- *Scoliosis*, a lateral and rotational curvature of the spine, can cause alterations in the structure of the pelvis and chest. It may be nonstructural, related to some other deformity or underlying problem, or structural, with changes in the spine and vertebrae because of congenital or other disorders. It is idiopathic in 70% to 80% of cases.
- *Spina bifida*, a neural tube defect, results in incomplete closure of the spine with the bones over the defect underdeveloped and unfused.
- Patients may have a combination, such as scoliokyphosis.

Scoliosis

Scoliosis is a lateral curvature of the spine that may be congenital, related to neuromuscular diseases, or idiopathic:

- *Congenital:* Part of the bony spine forms improperly or fuses during fetal development resulting in curvature, which may be slight or extensive.
- *Neuromuscular:* Neuropathic causes include those disorders involving upper motor neurons (cerebral palsy, spinal cord injury) and lower motor neurons (poliomyelitis, spinal muscular atrophy). Myopathic causes include muscular dystrophies. The pathophysiology of neuromuscular scoliosis remains unclear but may be related to muscle weakness; however, there is no consistent pattern of scoliosis related to spasticity, flaccidity, or weakness.
- *Idiopathic:* The pathophysiology is not yet clear but there appears to be a genetic component, which may involve multiple genes as severity of the disorder may vary widely within a family. There are 3 types: infantile (younger than 3 years of age) usually resolves but may progress; juvenile (ages 3 to 9 years) usually progresses and requires surgery; adolescent (ages 11 to 17) is the most common and affects females more than males. Curvature usually stabilizes.

Spinal Fusion

Spinal fusion is done to repair vertebral abnormalities, some resulting in spinal curvature of the spine with disability and deformity that can impair cardiopulmonary function and cause death. While exercises, braces, and electrical stimulation are used to treat mild conditions, surgical correction is often required:

- Spinal fusion usually includes spinal realignment and straightening with vertebrae fused together with bone grafts, usually from the child's iliac crest or a donor.
- The grafts may be placed posteriorly or anteriorly, often with the addition of instrumentation (hardware) in the form of rods, screws, wires, hooks, plates, and cages to stabilize and align vertebrae during fusion.
- A posterior fusion is done with a vertical incision along the length of the spine to be fused.
- An anterior fusion requires an incision will be back to front on one side of the rib cage (thoracic repair) or across rib cage and down the abdomen (for thoracic and lumbar repair).
- Endoscopic surgery may be done through small incisions.

Intracranial/Intraventricular Hemorrhage

SAH

Subarachnoid hemorrhage (SAH) may occur after trauma but is common from rupture of a berry aneurysm or an AVM. However, there are a number of disorders that may be implicated: neoplasms, sickle cell disease, infection, hemophilia, and leukemia. The first presenting symptom may be complaints of severe headache, nausea and vomiting, nuchal rigidity, palsy related to cranial nerve compression, retinal hemorrhages, and papilledema. Late complications include hyponatremia and hydrocephalus.

Symptoms worsen as intracranial pressure rises. SAH from aneurysm is classified as follows:

- Grade I: No symptoms or slight headache and nuchal rigidity.
- Grade II: Moderate to severe headache with nuchal rigidity and cranial nerve palsy.
- Grade III: Drowsy, progressing to confusion or mild focal deficits.
- Grade IV: Stupor, with hemiparesis (moderate to severe), early decerebrate rigidity, and vegetative disturbances.
- Grade V: Coma state with decerebrate rigidity.

Treatment includes: Identifying and treating underlying cause. Observing for re-bleeding; Anti-seizure medications (such as Dilantin®) to control seizures; antihypertensives; surgical repair if indicated.

Hemorrhages

Epidural

Hemorrhage is always a concern with head trauma because even injuries that appear slight can result in vascular rupture, resulting in hemorrhage between the skull and the brain. There are two types of hemorrhage that often occur from head trauma: epidural and subdural. Epidural hemorrhage is bleeding between the dura and the skull, pushing the brain downward and inward. The hemorrhage is usually caused by arterial tears, so bleeding is often rapid, leading to severe neurological deficits and respiratory arrest. Initially, the body compensates by rapidly absorbing cerebrospinal fluid and decreasing blood flow, but the compensatory measure is soon overwhelmed. The most common site is the parietotemporal region, forcing the medial part of the temporal lobe under the tentorial edge, compressing nerves and vessels. This type of injury usually results from skull fractures with middle meningeal artery lacerations or venous bleeding, such as those that occur with a blow to the head from a fall or motor vehicle accident.

Subdural Hemorrhage

Subdural hemorrhage is bleeding between the dura and the cerebrum, usually from tears in the cortical veins of the subdural space. It tends to develop more slowly than epidural hemorrhage and can result in a subdural hematoma. If the bleeding is acute and develops within minutes or hours of injury, the prognosis is poor. Subacute hematomas that develop more slowly cause varying degrees of injury. Subdural hemorrhage is a common injury related to trauma but it can result from coagulopathies or aneurysms. Symptoms of acute injury may occur within 24 to 48 hours, but subacute bleeding may not be evident for up to 2 weeks after injury. Chronic hemorrhage occurs primarily in elderly persons. Symptoms vary and may include bradycardia, tachycardia, hypertension, and alterations in consciousness. Older children and adults usually require surgical evacuation of the hematoma.

Seizure Disorders

Seizures are sudden involuntary abnormal electrical disturbances in the brain that can manifest as alterations of consciousness, spastic tonic and clonic movements, convulsions, and loss of consciousness. Seizures may be partial, affecting part of the brain, or generalized, affecting the whole brain. Seizures are a symptom of underlying pathology. Many seizures are transient. Some seizures may result from pathology, such as meningitis, cerebral edema, brain trauma, or brain tumors. Others are idiopathic, predisposing the person to recurrent seizures, usually of the same type. Seizures are believed to be caused by cells known as epileptogenic focus, which increase electrical discharge in response to physiological changes, such as fatigue or changes in blood sugar level. The electrical discharge spreads to the brainstem, causing generalized seizures. Seizures are characterized as focal (localized), focal with rapid generalization (spreading), and generalized (widespread). Seizure disorders with onset in childhood (younger than 4 years of age) usually cause more neurological damage than those that have a later onset.

Partial Seizures

Partial seizures are caused by an electrical discharged to a localized area of the cerebral cortex, such as the frontals, temporal, or parietal lobes, with seizure characteristics related to area of involvement. They may begin in a focal area and become generalized, often preceded by an aura.

- *Simple partial*: Unilateral motor symptoms including somatosensory, psychic, and autonomic.
    - Aversive: Eyes and head turned away from focal side
    - Sylvan (usually during sleep): Tonic-clonic movements of the face, salivation, and arrested speech.
- *Special sensory*: Various sensations (numbness, tingling, prickling, or pain) spreading from one area. May include visual sensations, posturing or hypertonia. Rare in children younger than 8 years.
- *Complex (Psychomotor)*: No loss of consciousness, but altered consciousness and nonresponsive with amnesia. May involve complex sensorium with bad tastes, auditory or visual hallucinations, feeling of déjà vu, strong fear. May carry out repetitive activities, such as walking, running, smacking lips, chewing, or drawling. Rarely aggressive. Seizure usually followed by prolonged drowsiness and confusion. Occurs age 3 through adolescence.

Generalized Seizures

Generalized seizures lack a focal onset and appear to involve both hemispheres, usually presenting with loss of consciousness and no preceding aura.

- Tonic-clonic (grand mal): Occurs without warning.
    - Tonic period (10 to 30 seconds): Eyes roll upward with loss of consciousness, arms flexed, stiffen in symmetric tonic contraction of body, apneic with cyanosis and salivating.
    - Clonic period (10 seconds to 30 minutes, but usually 30 seconds). Violent rhythmic jerking with contraction and relaxation. May be incontinent of urine and feces. Contractions slow and then stop.

Following seizures, there may be confusion, disorientation, and impairment of motor activity, speech, and vision for several hours. Headache, nausea, and vomiting may occur. Person often falls asleep and awakens conscious.

- *Absence (petit mal): Onset between* 4 and 12 years of age and usually ends in puberty. Onset is abrupt with brief loss of consciousness for 5 to 10 seconds and slight loss of muscle tone but often appears to be daydreaming. Lip smacking or eye twitching may occur.

Status Epilepticus

Status epilepticus (SE) is usually generalized tonic-clonic seizures that are characterized by a series of seizures with intervening time too short for regaining of consciousness. The constant assault and periods of apnea can lead to exhaustion, respiratory failure with hypoxemia and hypercapnia, cardiac failure, and death. There are a number of causes of SE:

- uncontrolled epilepsy or noncompliance with anticonvulsants
- infections, such as encephalitis; encephalopathy or brain attack
- drug toxicity (isoniazid); brain trauma
- Neoplasms; metabolic disorders.

Treatment includes:

- Anticonvulsants usually beginning with fast-acting benzodiazepine (lorazepam), often in steps, with administration of medication every 5 minutes until seizures subside.
- If cause is undetermined, acyclovir and ceftriaxone may be administered.
- If there is no response to the first 2 doses of anticonvulsants (refractory SE), rapid sequence intubation (RSI), which involves sedation and paralytic anesthesia, may be done while therapy continues. Combining phenobarbital and benzodiazepine can cause apnea, so intubation may be necessary.
- Phenytoin and phenobarbital are added.

Space-Occupying Lesions

Brain Tumors

Any type of brain tumor can occur in children and adults but the most common in children are those that arise from immature (blast) cells or supportive (glial) tissue:

- *Astrocytoma:* This arises from astrocytes, which are glial cells. It is the most common type of tumor, occurring throughout the brain but most common in the cerebellum of children. There are many types of astrocytomas, and most are slow growing. Some are operable while others are not. Radiation may be given after removal. Astrocytomas include glioblastomas, aggressively malignant tumors occurring most often in adults 45 to 70 years of age.
- *Brain stem glioma:* This may be fast or slow growing but is generally not operable because of location, although it may be treated with radiation or chemotherapy.
- *Craniopharyngioma:* This is a congenital, slow-growing, and benign cystic tumor but difficult to resect, and treated with surgery and radiation. They may be recurrent, especially if greater than 5 cm.
- *Meningioma:* Slow-growing meningeal tumor usually benign and occurring in women; surgically removed if causing symptoms.
- *Ependymoma:* This is usually benign in a cerebral hemisphere. Surgical excision and radiation are done.
- *Ganglioglioma:* This can occur anywhere in the brain but 70% occur above the tentorium (the membrane separating the cerebellum from the occipital lobes) in children. They are usually slow growing and benign.

- *Medulloblastoma:* There are many types of medulloblastoma, most arising in the cerebellum. They are malignant and fast growing. Surgical excision is done and often followed by radiation and chemotherapy, although recent studies show using just chemotherapy controls recurrence with less neurological damage.
- *Oligodendroglioma:* This tumor most often occurs in the cerebrum, primarily the frontal or temporal lobes, involving the myelin sheath of the neurons. It is slow growing and most common in those 40 to 60 years of age.
- *Optical nerve glioma:* This slow-growing tumor of the optic nerve is usually a form of astrocytoma. It is often associated with neurofibromatosis type I (NF1). Fifteen to forty percent of children with NF1 have optical nerve glioma. Despite surgical, chemotherapy or radiotherapy treatment, it is usually fatal.

ENCEPHALOPATHY

HYPERTENSIVE ENCEPHALOPATHY

Hypertensive encephalopathy can occur as part of hypertensive crisis. With chronic hypertension, the brain adapts to higher pressures to regulate blood flow, but in a hypertensive crisis, autoregulation of the blood-brain barrier is overwhelmed and the capillaries leak fluid into the tissue. Vasodilation takes place with resultant cerebral edema. Damage to arterioles occurs, causing increasing neurological deficits and papilledema. Hypertensive encephalopathy is relatively rare, but carries a high mortality rate and is most common in middle-aged men with long-standing hypertension. Symptoms usually develop over 1 to 2 days and include:

- nonspecific neurological deficits, such as weakness and visual abnormalities
- alterations in mental status, including confusion
- headache, often constant
- nausea and vomiting
- seizures
- coma

Hypertensive encephalopathy with cerebral edema requires prompt treatment in order to prevent neurological damage. *Treatment* includes identifying and treating the underlying causes for the hypertensive crisis and taking steps to lower the blood pressure:

- *Nitroprusside sodium (Nitropress®)* is usually used initially to lower BP.
- *Positioning* of patient to prevent obstruction of venous return from the head.
- *Monitoring blood gas* and maintaining $PaCO_2$ at 33 to 37 mm Hg to facilitate vasoconstriction of cerebral arteries.
- *Preventing hyperthermia* with antipyretics and cooling devices.
- *BP monitoring* and maintenance.
- *Seizure control* with phenobarbital and/or phenytoin.
- *Lidocaine* through endotracheal tube or intravenously prior to nasotracheal suctioning.
- *Diuretics*, such as osmotic agents (mannitol) and loop diuretics (furosemide), to control fluid volume.
- *Controlling metabolic demand* by measures to increase pain control and reduce stimulation.
- *Barbiturates* (pentobarbital, thiopental) in high doses may be used if other treatments fail to decrease intracranial pressure.

METABOLIC ENCEPHALOPATHY

Metabolic encephalopathy (hepatic encephalopathy) is damage to the brain resulting from a disturbance in metabolism, primarily hepatic failure to remove toxins from the blood. There may impairment in cerebral blood flow, cerebral edema, or increased intracranial pressure. It can occur as the result of ingestion of drugs or toxins, which can have a direct toxic affect on neurons, but can also occur with liver disease, especially when stressed by comorbidities, such as hemorrhage, hypoxemia, surgery, trauma, renal failure with dialysis, or electrolyte imbalances. *Symptoms* may vary:

- irritability and agitation
- alterations in consciousness
- dysphonia
- lack of coordination, spasticity
- seizures are common and may be the presenting symptom
- disorientation progressing to coma.

Prompt diagnosis is important because the condition may be reversible if underlying causes are identified and treated before permanent neuronal damage occurs. *Treatment* varies according to the underlying cause.

INFECTIOUS ENCEPHALOPATHY

Infectious encephalopathy is an encompassing term describing encephalopathies caused by a wide range of bacteria, viruses, or prions. Common to all infections are altered brain function that results in alterations in consciousness and personality, cognitive impairment, and lethargy. A wide range of neurological symptoms may occur: myoclonus, seizures, dysphagia, and dysphonia, neuromuscular impairment with muscle atrophy and tremors or spasticity. Treatment depends on the underlying cause and response to treatment. Prior infections are not treatable, but bacterial infections may respond to antibiotic therapy and viral infections may be self-limiting. HIV-related encephalopathy results from opportunistic infections as immune responses decrease, usually indicated by CD4 counts of less than 50. Aggressive antiretroviral treatment and treatment of the infection may reverse symptoms if permanent damage has not occurred for HIV-related encephalopathy. Treatment for other infectious encephalopathies varies according to the type of infection and underlying causes.

HEAD TRAUMA

IMPLICATIONS OF HEAD TRAUMA

Head trauma can occur as the result from intentional or unintentional blunt or penetrating trauma, such as from falls, automobile accidents, sports injuries, or violence. The degree of injury correlates with the impact force. The skull provides protection to the brain, but a severe blow can cause significant neurological damage.

- *Acceleration-deceleration injuries* are those in which a blow to the stationary head causes the elastic skull to change shape, pushing against the brain, which moves sharply backward in response, striking against the skull.
- *Bruising* can occur at the point of impact (*coup*) and the point where the brain hits the skull (*contrecoup*), so a blow to the frontal area can cause damage to the occipital region.
- *Shear injuries*, where vessels are torn, results from sudden movement of the brain.
- *Severe compression* may force the brain through the tentorial opening, damaging the brainstem.

Head injuries that occur at the time of trauma include fractures, contusions, hematomas, and diffuse cerebral and vascular injury. These injuries may result in hypoxia, increased intracranial pressure, and cerebral edema. Open injuries may result in infection. Patients often suffer initial hypertension, which increases intracranial pressure, decreasing perfusion. Often the primary problem with head trauma is a significant increase in swelling, which also interferes with perfusion, causing hypoxia and hypercapnia, which trigger increased blood flow. This increased volume at a time when injury impairs autoregulation increases cerebral edema, which, in turn, increases intracranial pressure and results in a further decrease in perfusion with resultant ischemia. If pressure continues to rise, the brain may herniate. Concomitant hypotension may result in hypoventilation, further complicating treatment.

Concussions, Contusions, and Lacerations

A variety of different injuries can occur as a result of head trauma:

- *Concussions* are the most common injury and are usually relatively transient, causing no permanent neurological damage. They may result in confusion, disorientation, and mild amnesia, but last only minutes or hours.
- *Contusions/Lacerations* are bruising and tears of cerebral tissue. There may be petechial areas at the impact site (coup) or larger bruising. Contrecoup injuries are less common in children than in adults. Areas most impacted by contusions and lacerations are the occipital, frontal, and temporal lobes. The degree of injury relates to the amount of vascular damage, but initial symptoms are similar to concussion; however, symptoms persist and may progress, depending upon the degree of injury. Lacerations are often caused by fractures.

Skull Fractures

Fractures are a common cause of penetrating wounds from bone fragments that cause cerebral lacerations. Open fractures are those in which the dura is torn, and closed is when the dura remain intact. While fractures by themselves do not cause neurological damage, force is needed to fracture the skull, often causing damage to underlying structures. Meningeal arteries lie in grooves on the underside of the skull, and a fracture can cause an arterial tear and hemorrhage. Skull fractures include:

- *Basilar:* Occurs in bones at the base of the brain and can cause severe brainstem damage.
- *Comminuted:* Skull fractures into small pieces.
- *Compound:* Surface laceration extends to a skull fracture.
- *Depressed:* Pieces of the skull are depressed inward on the brain tissue, often producing dural tears.
- *Linear/Hairline:* Skull fracture forms a thin line without any splintering.

Neurologic Infectious Diseases

Bacterial Meningitis

Bacterial meningitis may be caused by a wide range of pathogenic organisms, with the predominant agents varying with age:

- 1 month or younger; Escherichia coli, group B streptococci, Listeria monocytogenes, and Neisseria meningitidis.
- 1 to 2 months: group B streptococci.
- Older than 2 months: *Streptococcus pneumoniae, N. meningitidis.* Unvaccinated (Hib vaccine) children are at risk for *Haemophilus influenzae.* These are most common in adults.

Bacterial infections usually arise from spread distant infections, although they can enter the CNS from surgical wounds, invasive devices, nasal colonization, or penetrating trauma. The infective process includes inflammation, exudates, white blood cell accumulation, and tissue damage with the brain showing evidence of hyperemia and edema. Purulent exudate covers the brain and invades and blocks the ventricles, obstructing cerebrospinal fluid (CSF) and leading to increased intracranial pressure. Since antibodies specific to bacteria do not cross the blood-brain barrier, the body's ability to fight the infection is very poor. Diagnosis is usually based on lumbar puncture examination of CSF and symptoms.

West Nile Virus

West Nile virus is an RNA virus, spread by infected mosquitoes. Infection has been traced to donor organs, blood transfusions, and breast milk, although the blood supply has been monitored for WNV since 2003. While West Nile virus is more common in adults, especially elderly persons, it can affect infants and children, who show symptoms more readily than adults. The incubation period ranges from 2 to 14 days. There are 4 types of infection:

- *Viremia*: 80%, infection but no symptoms.
- *Mild*: 20% (West Nile fever), characterized by fever, malaise, lymphadenopathy, headache, rash, nausea, and vomiting. The acute stage is usually is self-limiting within a few days, but symptoms can persist for weeks, and include muscular weakness, fatigue, concentration problems, fever, and headache. About 30% require hospitalization.
- *Severe*: Less than 1%, severe neurological symptoms with meningitis and associated symptoms being the most common in children and younger adults.
- *West Nile poliomyelitis*: Acute flaccid paralysis can result in respiratory arrest and death.

Treatment is supportive during illness and preventive (insect repellant).

ARBOVIRUSES

There are a number of arboviruses in addition to West Nile virus that can cause flu-like symptoms that progress to viral encephalitis, and incidence is increasing across the United States, often spread by mosquitoes. Because many people are unaware of emerging causes for diseases, the cause of the ensuing encephalitis is frequently misdiagnosed. Encephalitis is an infection of the brain tissue and usually lasts for 2 to 3 weeks. *Symptoms* vary somewhat from one type of infection to another, but they have similar characteristics.

- Onset usually involves flu-like symptoms with sore throat, headaches, muscle aches, fever and chills, myalgia. In some cases, a rash may appear.
- Progressive symptoms include photophobia, vomiting, and increased weakness.
- Advanced symptoms may include altered mental status, seizures, memory loss, coma, and death.

Encephalitis may also result from complications of Lyme disease, spread by infected ticks. One of the most common causes of encephalitis is the herpes simplex virus.

ARBOVIRAL ENCEPHALITIDES

Arboviral encephalitides include:

- *Eastern equine encephalitis* (EEE) (Togaviridae) has a high mortality rate and is most common in the eastern and gulf coast areas of the United States. Sporadic outbreaks occur. Half of survivors have residual neurological damage, especially children.
- *Western equine encephalitis (WEE)* (Togaviridae) is similar to EEE but found on the West Coast and the Midwest.
- *Venezuelan equine encephalitis* (Togaviridae) occurs primarily in Florida and southwest United States.
- St. Louis encephalitis (Flaviviridae) occurs throughout the United States but most infections are subclinical; however, if symptoms are present, about 50% of those younger than 20 years of age develop encephalitis and 5% to 15% die.
- *La Cross encephalitis* (Bunyaviridae) is scattered and rare and usually results in mild disease with mortality rate less than 1%.
- *Cache Valley virus* (Bunyaviridae) has occurred in the Southeast and Wisconsin and is believed to be underreported. It occurs primarily in children younger than 16 years of age. Mortality rates are less than 1% but neurological damage may persist.

BACTERIAL MENINGITIS

Bacterial meningitis may manifest differently, depending upon the age of the person:

- *Neonates*: Signs may be very nonspecific, such as weight loss, hypo- or hyperthermia, jaundice, irritability, lethargy, or irregular respirations with periods of apnea. More specific signs may include increasing signs of illness, difficulty feeding with loss of suck reflex, hypotonia, weak cry, seizures, and bulging fontanels (may be a late sign). Nuchal rigidity does not usually occur with neonates.
- *Infants and young children*: Classic symptoms usually do not appear until 2 years of age or older. Signs may include fever, poor feeding, vomiting, irritability, and bulging fontanel. Nuchal rigidity in some children.
- *Older children and adolescents/adults:* Abrupt onset, including fever, chills, headache, and alterations of consciousness with seizures, agitation, and irritability. May have photophobia, hallucinations, aggressive behavior, or stuporous and lapsing into coma. Nuchal rigidity progressing to opisthotonos. Reflexes are variable but positive Kernig and Brudzinski signs. Signs may relate to particular bacteria, such as rashes, sore joints, or draining ear.

INFECTION CONTINUUM

There are a number of terms used to refer to **severe infections** and they are often used interchangeably, but they are part of a continuum:

- *Bacteremia* is the present of bacteria in the blood but without systemic infection.
- *Septicemia* is a systemic infection caused by pathogens (usually bacteria or fungi) present in the blood.
- *Systemic inflammatory response syndrome (SIRS)* is a generalized inflammatory response affecting may organ systems, and may be caused by infectious or noninfectious agents, such as trauma, burns, adrenal insufficiency, pulmonary embolism, and drug overdose. If an infectious agent is identified or suspected, SIRS is an aspect of sepsis. Infective agents include a wide range of bacteria and fungi, including *Streptococcus pneumoniae* and *Staphylococcus aureus.* SIRS includes 2 of the following:
    - elevated (greater than 38°C) or subnormal rectal temperature (less than 36°C)
    - tachypnea or $PaCO_2$ less than 32 mm Hg
    - tachycardia
    - leukocytosis (greater than 12,000) or leukopenia (less than 4,000).

Infections can progress from bacteremia, septicemia, and SIRS to the following:

Sepsis is presence of infection either locally or systemically in which there is a generalized life-threatening inflammatory response (SIRS). It includes all the indications for SIRS as well as one of the following:

- changes in mental status
- hypoxemia (less than 72 mm Hg) without pulmonary disease
- elevation in plasma lactate
- decreased urinary output less than 5 mL/kg/wt for at least 1 hour.

Severe sepsis includes both indications of SIRS and sepsis as well as indications of increasing organ dysfunction with inadequate perfusion and/or hypotension.

Septic shock is a progression from severe sepsis in which refractory hypotension occurs despite treatment. There may be indications of lactic acidosis.

Multiorgan dysfunction syndrome (MODS) is the most common cause of sepsis-related death. Cardiac function becomes depressed, acute respiratory distress syndrome (ARDS) may develop, and renal failure may follow acute tubular necrosis or cortical necrosis. Thrombocytopenia appears in about 30% of those affected and may result in disseminated intravascular coagulation (DIC). Liver damage and bowel necrosis may occur.

Multiorgan Dysfunction Syndrome

MODS is progressive deterioration and failure of 2 or more organ systems with mortality rates of 45% to 50% with 2 organ systems involved and up to 80% to 100% if there are at least 3 systems failing. Trauma patients and those with severe conditions, such as shock, burns, and sepsis, are particularly vulnerable, especially in those older than 65 years of age. MODS may be primary or secondary:

- ***Primary*** MODS relates to direct injury/disorder of the organ systems, resulting in dysfunction, such as with thermal injuries, traumatic pulmonary injuries, and invasive infections.
- ***Secondary*** MODS relates to dysfunction of organ systems not directly involved in injury/disorder but developing as the result of SIRS as the patient's immune and inflammatory responses become dysregulated. In some patients, failure of organ systems is sequential, usually progressing from the lungs, the liver, the GI system, and the kidneys to the heart. However, in other cases, various organ systems may fail at the same time.

Neuromuscular Disorders

Facioscapulohumeral and Limb-Girdle Muscular Dystrophy

Muscular dystrophies are genetic disorders with gradual degeneration of muscle fibers and progressive weakness and atrophy of skeletal muscles and loss of mobility. Types differ according to the muscles involved, the age of onset, and the speed of progression:

- ***Facioscapulohumeral muscular dystrophy*** (Landouzy-Dejerine) is a slowly progressive autosomal recessive disorder with onset usually between 10 and 24 years of age. Typically, the shoulders angle forward, the face loses mobility, and the child cannot raise the arms above the head because of weakness of the upper arms. The lower extremities may be affected as the disease progresses.
- ***Limb-girdle muscular dystrophy*** is a group of autosomal recessive or dominant disorders with onset in later childhood or adolescence, manifesting as weakness of proximal muscles of the pelvic and shoulder girdles although muscles in proximity to these (upper arms and thighs) may weaken over time. There are over a dozen forms, related to specific genetic defects. Some forms cause serious disability in a few years and others progress very slowly.

Duchenne

Pseudohypertrophic (Duchenne) muscular dystrophy is the most common form and the most severe. It is an X-linked disorder in about 50% of the cases with the rest sporadic mutations, affecting males almost exclusively. An abnormal cycloskeletal protein (dystrophin) causes the sarcolemma (membrane) of the muscle to allow excess calcium, which in turn leads to muscle necrosis. Children typically have some delay in motor development, with difficulty walking and have evidence of muscle weakness by about the age of 3 years. Pseudohypertrophic refers to enlargement of muscles by fatty infiltration associated with muscular atrophy, which causes contractures and deformities of joints. Abnormal bone development results in spinal and other skeletal deformities. The disease progresses rapidly, and most children are wheelchair-bound by about 12 years of age. As the disease progresses, it involves the muscles of the diaphragm and other muscles needed for respiration. Mild to frank mental deficiency is common. Facial, oropharyngeal, and respiratory muscles weaken late in the disease. Cardiomegaly commonly occurs.

Guillain-Barré Syndrome

Guillain-Barré syndrome (GBS) is an autoimmune disorder of the myelinated motor peripheral nervous system, often triggered by a viral gastroenteritis or *Campylobacter jejuni* infection. *Symptoms* include: numbness and tingling with increasing weakness of lower extremities that may become generalized, sometimes resulting in complete paralysis and inability to breathe without ventilatory support. Deep tendon reflexes are typically absent and some people experience facial weakness and ophthalmoplegia (paralysis of muscles controlling movement of eyes). *Diagnosis* is by history, clinical symptoms, and lumbar puncture, which often shows increased protein with normal glucose and cell count although protein may not increase for a week or more. *Treatment* is supportive. Patients should be hospitalized for observation and placed on ventilator support if forced vital capacity is less than 2 L. While there is no definitive treatment, plasma exchange or IV immunoglobulin shortens the duration of symptoms.

Review Video: Guillain-Barre Syndrome
Visit mometrix.com/academy and enter code: 742900

MYASTHENIA GRAVIS

Myasthenia gravis (MG) is an autoimmune disorder of the neuromuscular system in which acetylcholine receptors are damaged at neural synapses, preventing transmission of impulses to contract muscles. The thymus gland develops abnormalities and sometimes thymoma. *Symptoms* of MG include muscle weakness, which decreases with rest. Eye muscles are often affected first, resulting in ptosis and visual disturbances such as diplopia. General weakness in extremities, neck, and face, as well as dysphagia and slurred speech occur. Acute respiratory failure can occur as part of *myasthenic crisis* before diagnosis or be related to fever, infection, or drug therapy. *Diagnosis* of MG is from history, neurological exam, antibody testing, edrophonium chloride testing to differentiate exacerbation of disease from cholinergic crisis, electromyogram, and pulmonary function tests. *Treatments*:

- Crisis: Mechanical ventilation and treatment of underlying cause.
- Thymectomy: Relieves symptoms in 70%.
- Immunosuppressants: azathioprine, cyclosporine, and prednisone.
- Acetylcholinesterase inhibitors: pyridostigmine.

Many drugs can trigger respiratory failure, so drug lists should be checked and ventilatory equipment available when treating MG patients.

PARKINSON'S DISEASE

Parkinson's disease (PD) is an extrapyramidal movement motor system disorder caused by loss of brain cells that produce dopamine. Typical *symptoms* include tremor of face and extremities, rigidity, bradykinesia, akinesia, poor posture, and lack of balance and coordination, causing increasing problems with mobility, talking, and swallowing. Some patients may suffer depression, mood changes, and dementia. Tremors usually present unilaterally in an upper extremity. *Diagnosis* includes:

- Cogwheel rigidity test: Extremity put through passive range of motion causes increased muscle tone and ratchet-like movements.
- Physical and neurological exam.
- Complete history to rule out drug-induced Parkinson's akinesia.

Treatment includes:

- Symptomatic support.
- Dopaminergic therapy: levodopa, amantadine, and carbidopa.
- Anticholinergics: trihexyphenidyl, benztropine.
- Drug-induced Parkinson's disease: Terminate drugs.

Drug therapy tends to decrease in efficiency over time, and patients may present with marked increase in symptoms. Discontinuing the drugs for 1 week may exacerbate symptoms initially, but functioning may improve when drugs are reintroduced.

MULTIPLE SCLEROSIS

Multiple sclerosis is an autoimmune disorder of the CNS in which the myelin sheath around the nerves is damaged and replaced by scar tissue that prevents conduction of nerve impulses. Symptoms vary widely and can include problems with balance and coordination, tremors, slurring of speech, cognitive impairment, vision impairment and nystagmus, pain, and bladder and bowel dysfunction. Symptoms may be relapsing-remitting, progressive, or a combination. Onset is usually at 20 to 30 years of age, with incidence higher in females. Patient may initially present with problems walking or falling or optic neuritis (30%), causing loss of central vision. Males may complain of sexual dysfunction as an early symptom. Others have dysuria with urinary retention. Diagnosis is based on clinical and neurological examination and MRI. Treatment is symptomatic and includes treatment to shorten duration of episodes and slow progress.

Glucocorticoids: Methylprednisolone.
Immunomodulator: Interferon beta, glatiramer acetate, natalizumab.
Immunosuppressant: Mitoxantrone.
Hormone: Estriol (for females).

Hydrocephalus

The ventricular system produces and circulates cerebrospinal fluid (CSF). There are right and left lateral ventricles, which open into the third ventricle at the interventricular foramen (foramen of Monro). The aqueduct of Sylvius connects the third and fourth ventricles. The fourth ventricle, anterior to the cerebellum, supplies CSF to the subarachnoid space and the spinal cord (dorsal surface). The CSF circulates and then returns to the brain and is absorbed in the arachnoid villi. Hydrocephalus occurs when there is an imbalance between production and absorption of CSF in the ventricles, resulting from impaired absorption or obstruction, which may be congenital or acquired. There are 2 common types of hydrocephalus:

- *Communicating*: CSF flows (communicates) between the ventricles but is not absorbed in the subarachnoid space (arachnoid villi).
- *Noncommunicating*: CSF is obstructed (noncommunicating) between the ventricles with obstruction, often stenosis of the aqueduct of Sylvius, but it can occur anywhere in the system.

Symptoms of **hydrocephalus** depend on the age of onset. In *early infancy*, before closure of cranial sutures, head enlargement is the most common presentation, but in adults with less elasticity in the skull, neurological symptoms usually relate to increasing pressure on structures of the brain. Hydrocephalus may occur at any age, but the type that occurs in *younger or middle-aged adults* is different than that common in children or those older than 50 years of age. Hydrocephalus in younger and middle-aged adults may result from a congenital defect, hydrocephalus of infancy with shunt failure, or trauma, and is characterized by:

- headache relieved by vomiting, papilledema
- lack of bladder control
- strabismus and other visual disorders
- ataxia
- irritability
- lethargy
- confusion and impairment of cognitive abilities.

With *adult-onset normal pressure hydrocephalus* (older than 50 years of age), CSF increases and dilates the ventricles, but frequently without increasing intracranial pressure. The cause is often unclear. Symptoms include gait disturbance, bladder control issues, and mild dementia. *Treatment* for all types of hydrocephalus involves shunting and relieving pressure.

Hydrocephalus is diagnosed through CT and MRI, which help to determine the cause. Treatment may vary somewhat depending upon the underlying disorder, which may require treatment. For example, if obstruction is caused by a tumor, surgical excision to directly remove the obstruction is required. Generally, however, most hydrocephalus is treated with shunts:

- *Ventriculoperitoneal shunt*: This procedure is the most common and consists of placement of a ventricular catheter directly into the ventricles (usually lateral) at one end with the other end in the peritoneal area to drain away excess CSF. There is a one-way valve near the proximal end that prevents backflow but opens when pressure rises to drain fluid. In some cases the distal end drains into the right atrium.
- *Third ventriculostomy*: A small opening is made in the base of the third ventricle so CSF can bypass an obstruction. This procedure is not common and is done with a small endoscope.

Acute Spinal Cord Injury

Spinal Cord Injuries

Spinal cord injury (SCI) may result from blunt trauma (such as an automobile accident), a fall from a height, sports injuries, and penetrating trauma (such as a gunshot or knife wound). Damage results from mechanical injury and secondary responses resulting from hemorrhage, edema, and ischemia. The type of symptoms relate to the area and degree of injury:

- *Anterior cord:* The posterior column functions remain, so there is sensation of touch, vibration, and position remaining below injury but with complete paralysis and loss of sensations of pain and temperature. Prognosis is poor.
- *Brown-Séquard:* The cord is hemisected, resulting in spastic paresis, loss of sense of position and vibration on the injured side, and loss of pain and temperature on the other side. Prognosis is good.

Spinal cord injuries include:

- *Cauda equina*: Damage is below L1 with variable loss of motor ability and sensation, and bowel and bladder dysfunction. Injury is to peripheral nerves, which can regenerate, so prognosis is better than for other lesions of the spinal cord.
- *Central cord:* Results from hyperextension and ischemia or stenosis of cervical spine, causing quadriparesis (more severe in upper extremities) with some loss of sensations of pain and temperature. Prognosis is good, but fine motor skills are often impaired in upper extremities.
- *Conus medullaris*: Injury to lower spine (lower lumbar and sacral nerves).
- *Posterior cord*: Motor function is preserved but without sensation.
- *Spinal shock:* Injury at T6 or above, results in flaccid paralysis below lesion with loss of sensations and rectal tone, bradycardia, and hypotension.

Patients with spinal cord injuries should immediately be evaluated for airway control, and the spine kept immobilized. *Treatment* includes:

- intubation and ventilation (usually with sedation) to prevent respiratory failure for injuries at C5 or above
- IV fluids to prevent and treat hypotension
- examination, blood cell count, chest x-ray, and abdominal ultrasound and/or lavage to evaluate blood loss
- complete neurological exam after patient is stabilized
- x-ray or CT scans
- MRI to examine nerve or ligamentous injury
- corticosteroids for neurological deficits from blunt trauma:
    - begin within 8 hours of injury
    - methylprednisolone 30 mg/kg bolus IV over 15 minutes
    - 45-minute break

  - methylprednisolone 5.4 mg/kg per hour for 23 hours
- surgical decompression as needed for penetrating wounds
- antibiotics as indicated for penetrating stab wounds
- nonoperative spinal stabilization as indicated.

NEUROGENIC SHOCK

Neurogenic shock occurs when injury to the CNS from trauma resulting in acute spinal cord injury (from both blunt and penetrating injuries, neurological diseases, drugs, or anesthesia) impairs the autonomic nervous system that controls the cardiovascular system. Symptoms include hypotension and warm, dry skin related to lack of vascular tone resulting in hypothermia from loss of cutaneous heat. Bradycardia is a common but not universal symptom. The degree of symptoms relates to the level of injury with injuries above T1 capable of causing disruption of the entire sympathetic nervous system and lower injuries causing various degrees of disruption. Even incomplete spinal cord injury can cause neurogenic shock.

Treatment includes:

- ABCDE (airway, breathing, circulation, disability evaluation, exposure)
- rapid fluid administration with crystalloid to keep mean arterial pressure at 85 to 90 mm Hg
- placement of pulmonary artery catheter to monitor fluid overload
- inotropes (dopamine, dobutamine) if fluids do not correct hypotension
- atropine for persistent bradycardia
- transfer to trauma unit or facility.

RESTLESS LEG SYNDROME

Restless leg syndrome (RLS) is characterized by pain and paresthesia in the legs at rest, especially in the evening and at night. Some people also have periodic jerking of limbs. The discomfort in the legs is relieved by moving the legs, but this often results in difficulty sleeping and resultant exhaustion during the daytime. Neurological examination is typically normal, but family history of RLS is common. In some cases, the symptoms may relate to iron deficiency anemia, so hemoglobin and hematocrit should be checked. *Treatment* includes:

- Ropinirole and pramipexole have been approved by the FDA specifically for RLS.
- Levodopa/carbidopa 25/100 mg sustained-release ½ tab at bedtime.
- Opioids: Propoxyphene, tramadol
- Cyclobenzaprine 10 mg at bedtime
- Anticonvulsants: Gabapentin 100 mg at bedtime
- Iron replacement therapy if indicated.

Some people have relief of symptoms if they reduce caffeine, alcohol, and tobacco use.

MARFAN SYNDROME

Marfan syndrome is a genetic disorder of the connective tissue. Connective tissue, such as tendons, ligaments, heart valves, and blood vessels, is often defective and weak. Depending upon the severity of the disorder, people diagnosed with this disorder may be restricted from strenuous activities, such as team sports, especially contact sports that may result in chest trauma, or isometric exercises, such as weightlifting. The patient with symptoms of Marfan syndrome should be referred to a specialist for assessment of aortic abnormalities. Traits can include:

- tall, thin stature with loose joints, with the long bones disproportionately long
- scoliosis
- flat feet
- pectus carinatum (pigeon chest) or pectus excavatum (funnel chest)

- long, narrow face with high arched roof of mouth and crowding of teeth
- dislocation of lenses of eyes and sometimes retinal detachment, myopia
- aortic dilatation (with risk of dissection)
- cardiac valve disorders with heart murmur
- stretch marks
- abdominal/inguinal hernia
- sleep apnea (rare).

Gastrointestinal

GI Abnormalities

Gastroesophageal Reflux Disease (GERD)

Gastroesophageal reflux disease (GERD) is involuntary regurgitation of stomach contents into the esophagus, usually caused by decreased tone in the gastroesophageal valve and hiatal hernia, causing damage to the mucosal lining of the esophagus. Chronic esophagitis, strictures, Barrett esophagus (abnormal changes in cells of distal esophagus), and esophageal cancer may develop. GERD *symptoms* include:

- epigastric pain and "heartburn," dysphagia
- chronic cough, especially at night, and hoarseness
- earache
- sinusitis.

Treatment includes:

- avoiding large meals or after-dinner snacking and eating at least 3 hours before going to bed or lying down
- modifying food intake to avoid coffee, alcohol, fatty food, spicy foods, and cruciferous vegetables
- sleeping with head of the bed elevated and on left side
- medications include histamine-2 receptor blockers (famotidine), proton pump inhibitors, alginic acid (Gaviscon®),, and antacids (without aluminum)
- surgical repair (fundoplication) may be needed if medical treatment is not adequate.

Diverticulosis and Diverticulitis

Diverticulosis is a condition in which diverticula (saclike pouches of the bowel lining that extend through a defect in the muscle layer) occur anywhere within the GI tract. Diverticulitis occurs as diverticula become inflamed when food or bacteria are retained within diverticula. This may result in abscess, obstruction, perforation, bleeding, or fistula. *Symptoms* are similar to appendicitis and include:

- steady pain in left lower quadrant (sigmoid diverticulitis)
- change in bowel habits
- tenesmus
- dysuria from irritation
- toxic reactions: fever, severe pain, leukocytosis
- recurrent urinary infections from fistula
- paralytic ileus from peritonitis or intra-abdominal irritation.

Diagnosis is per CT, as barium enema will show diverticula but not inflammation. *Treatment* includes:

- rehydration and electrolytes per intravenous fluids
- nothing by mouth initially
- antibiotics, broad spectrum (IV if toxic reactions)

- nasogastric (NG) suction if necessary for obstruction
- careful observation for signs of perforation or obstruction

Irritable Bowel Syndrome

Irritable bowel syndrome is a chronic disorder characterized by abdominal discomfort and change in bowel habits. It is more common in females (66%) than males and may be associated with depression and history of bacterial gastroenteritis. Symptoms are often vague but usually do not include sudden onset, fever, nocturnal diarrhea, or weight loss. Typical symptoms include:

- abdominal pain relieved by defecation
- change in frequency of defection, which may occur more frequently (greater than 3 times daily) or less frequently (less than 3 times weekly)
- change in character of stool from very hard to very loose and watery
- difficulty with defecation involving straining, urgency, or inability to completely evacuate rectum
- Abdominal distension.

Diagnosis is based on symptoms and laboratory tests to rule out other disorders (such as celiac disease). *Treatment* includes reducing stressors, dietary management (reducing fatty foods, caffeine, and foods that cause flatulence), medications (antispasmodics, antidiarrheals, laxatives, tricyclic antidepressants, serotonin receptor agonists and antagonists, nonabsorbable antibiotics [rifaximin 400 mg three times daily]), and cognitive therapy for relaxation.

Peritonitis

Peritonitis (inflammation of the peritoneum) may be primary (from infection of blood or lymph) or, more commonly, secondary, related to perforation or trauma of the GI tract. Common causes include perforated bowel, ruptured appendix, abdominal trauma, abdominal surgery, peritoneal dialysis or chemotherapy, or leakage of sterile fluids, such as blood, into the peritoneum.

Symptoms of peritonitis are those of an acute abdomen:

- diffuse abdominal pain with rebound tenderness (Blumberg sign)
- abdominal rigidity
- paralytic ileus
- fever (with infection)
- nausea and vomiting
- sinus tachycardia.

Diagnosis is made according to clinical presentation, abdominal x-rays, which may show distention of the intestines or air in the peritoneum, and laboratory findings, such as leukocytosis. Blood cultures may indicate sepsis. *Treatment* includes:

- IV fluids and electrolytes
- broad-spectrum antibiotics
- surgical consultation for laparoscopy as indicated to determine cause of peritonitis and effect repair.

Cholecystitis

Cholecystitis can result in obstruction of the bile duct related to calculi as well as pancreatitis from obstruction of the pancreatic duct. The disease is most common in overweight women 20 to 40 years of age but can occur in pregnant women and people of all ages, especially those who are diabetic or elderly. Children may develop cholecystitis secondary to cystic fibrosis, obesity, or total parenteral nutrition. *Symptoms* range from asymptomatic to severe right upper quadrant or epigastric pain, persisting 2 to 6 hours per episode. Disease of the biliary tract may cause radiation of pain to the back and nausea and vomiting. Cholangitis may result in jaundice and altered mental status. *Diagnosis* is confirmed by ultrasound, as laboratory findings may be within normal range. *Treatment* includes:

- antibiotics for sepsis or ascending cholangitis
- antispasmodic agents (glycopyrrolate) for biliary colic and vomiting
- analgesics (meperidine for acute pain)
- antiemetics (promethazine)
- surgical consultation to determine if laparoscopic or open cholecystectomy is warranted.

Esophageal Varices

Esophageal varices are torturous dilated veins in the submucosa of the esophagus (usually the distal portion), a complication of cirrhosis of the liver in which obstruction of the portal vein causes an increase in collateral vessels, a decrease in circulation to the liver, and an increase in pressure in the collateral vessels in the submucosa of the esophagus and stomach. This causes the vessels to dilate. Because they tend to be fragile and inelastic, they tear easily, causing sudden massive esophageal hemorrhage. Bleeding from varices occurs in 19% to 50% with associated mortality rates of 40% to 70%. *Treatment* may include:

- fluid and blood replacement
- IV vasopressin, somatostatin, and octreotide to decrease portal venous pressure and provide vasoconstriction
- endoscopic injection with sclerosing agents
- endoscopic variceal band ligation
- esophagogastric balloon tamponade to apply direct pressure
- transjugular intrahepatic portosystemic shunting (TIPS) creates a channel between systemic and portal venous systems to reduce portal hypertension. A variety of other shunts may be done surgically if bleeding persists.

Acute GI Hemorrhage

Acute Gastrointestinal Hemorrhage (Peptic Ulcers)

GI hemorrhage may occur in the upper or lower GI track. The primary cause (50% to 70%) of GI hemorrhage is peptic ulcer disease (gastric and duodenal ulcers), which results in deterioration of the gastric mucosal lining, compromising the glycoprotein mucous barrier and the gastroduodenal epithelial cells that provide protection from gastric secretions. The secretions literally digest the mucosal and submucosal layers, damaging blood vessels and causing hemorrhage. The primary causes are NSAIDs and infection with *Helicobacter pylori. Symptoms* include:

- abdominal pain and distention
- hematemesis
- bloody or tarry stools
- hypotension with tachycardia.

Treatment includes:

- fluid replacement with transfusions if necessary
- antibiotic therapy for *H. pylori*
- endoscopic thermal therapy to cauterize or injection therapy (hypertonic saline, epinephrine, ethanol) to cause vasoconstriction
- arteriography with intra-arterial infusion of vasopressin and/or embolizing agents, such as stainless steel coils, platinum microcoils, or Gelfoam pledgets vagotomy and pyloroplasty if bleeding persists.

Stress-Related Erosive Syndrome

Stress-related erosive syndrome (SRES) (stress ulcers) occurs most frequently in those who are critically ill, such as those with severe or multiorgan trauma, mechanical ventilation, sepsis, severe burns, and head injury with increased intracranial pressure. Stress induces changes in the gastric mucosal lining and decreased perfusion of the mucosa, causing ischemia. SRES involves hemorrhage in at least 30%, with mortality rates of 30% to 80%, so prompt identification and treatment is critical. The lesions tend to be diffuse, so they are more difficult to treat than peptic ulcers. *Symptoms* include:

- coffee-ground emesis
- hematemesis
- abdominal discomfort.

Treatment includes prophylaxis in those at risk:

- sucralfate (Carafate®) protects mucosa against pepsin
- famotidine (Pepcid®), nizatidine (Axid®), or cimetidine (Tagamet®) reduces gastric secretions.

Treatment for active bleeding includes:

- intra-arterial infusion of vasopressin
- intra-arterial embolization
- oversewing of ulcers or total gastrectomy if bleeding persists.

Bowel Infarction/Obstruction/Perforation

Chemical Trauma

Chemical trauma may be caused by leakage or incontinence of body fluids, such as urine, feces, and exudate, or chemicals applied to the skin, such as lotions, iodine, soap, organic solvents, acids, and adhesives. Reactions to irritant contact dermatitis may vary widely from an itching rash similar to allergic contact dermatitis to cracks and fissures in the skin, especially on the hands, or denudement of skin, often in the perineal area. The skin reaction may be rapid and extremely painful. *Treatment* includes:

- Identifying irritant and eliminating contact with skin.
- Gentle cleansing of skin to remove irritant but avoid further skin irritation.
- Use of skin sealants or skin barriers as indicated to protect the skin and allow healing.
- Use of appropriate skin care products and containment devices.
- Monitoring of dressings and periwound condition daily.

Bowel Obstruction and Infarction

Bowel obstruction occurs when there is a mechanical obstruction of the passage of intestinal contents because of constriction of the lumen, occlusion of the lumen, or lack of muscular contractions (paralytic ileus). Obstruction may be caused by congenital or acquired abnormalities/disorders. *Symptoms* include:

- abdominal pain and distention
- abdominal rigidity
- vomiting and dehydration
- diminished or no bowel sounds
- severe constipation (obstipation)
- respiratory distress from diaphragm pushing against pleural cavity
- shock as plasma volume diminishes and electrolytes enter intestines from bloodstream
- sepsis as bacteria proliferates in bowel and invade bloodstream.

Bowel infarction is ischemia of the intestines related to severely restricted blood supply. It can be the result of a number of different conditions, such as strangulated bowel or occlusion of arteries of the mesentery, and may follow untreated bowel obstruction. Patients present with acute abdomen and shock, and mortality rates are very high even with resection of infarcted bowel.

Intestinal Perforation

Intestinal perforation is a complete rupture or penetration of the intestinal wall. There are a number of causes:

- traumatic injuries, such as gunshot or knife wounds
- NSAIDs and/or aspirin, especially in elderly with diverticulitis
- acute appendicitis
- peptic ulcer disease
- Iatrogenic causes: laparoscopy, endoscopy, colonoscopy, radiotherapy
- bacterial infections
- inflammatory bowel diseases, such as Crohn's disease or ulcerative colitis
- ingestion of toxic substances (acids) or foreign bodies (toothpicks).

The danger posed by infection after perforation varies depending upon the site. The stomach and proximal portions of the small intestine have little bacteria, but the distal portion of the small intestine contains aerobic bacteria, such as *E. coli*, as well as anaerobic bacteria. *Symptoms* include abdominal pain and distention, and rigidity, fever, guarding and rebound tenderness, tachycardia, and paralytic ileus with nausea and vomiting. *Treatment* is as for peritonitis, with antibiotics and surgical repair.

Paralytic Ileus

Paralytic ileus is the lack of intestinal contractions and bowel sounds because of paralysis of the bowel caused by excessive manipulation during surgery (most common), prolonged period of anesthesia, infection (such as peritonitis and appendicitis), or narcotic pain medications. *Symptoms* resemble those of bowel obstruction, although the intestines remain patent:

- constipation and lack of flatulence
- Abdominal distension
- nausea and vomiting
- diffuse abdominal discomfort
- lack of bowel sounds on auscultation.

Patients should be encouraged to exercise and roll from side to side frequently to stimulate contractions. Ileus may require IV fluids and nasogastric tube to decompress the stomach and prevent vomiting until normal bowel activity returns. Oral foods/fluids should be avoided. Most cases resolve within a few days, but contrast studies should be done if the ileus is prolonged to rule out mechanical obstruction.

Adhesions

Adhesions occur when loops of intestine adhere to slow healing or scarred areas by bands of fibrous tissue after abdominal surgery, occurring in about 90%. While most cause no problems, adhesions can become obstructive. About 60% to 70% of small bowel obstructions in adults are caused by adhesions. While adhesions begin to develop quickly after surgery, adverse symptoms may not occur for years. In some cases, bands may encircle an intestinal segment, leading to ischemia. As adhesions pull on organs, pain develops. Typical *symptoms* include:

- pain with deep breath (if adhesions superior to the liver)
- pain during exercise
- intestinal obstruction (pain, distention)

- loose stools
- nausea and vomiting

Diagnosis is usually by laparoscopy, although CT scans may show the extent of adhesions and damage. *Treatment* may be symptomatic if symptoms are not acute, but severe symptoms may require laparoscopy or laparotomy to release adhesions.

Short Gut (Bowel) Syndrome

Short gut (bowel) syndrome occurs when removal of part of the small intestine results in a malabsorptive condition. *Symptoms* relate to the amount of bowel removed and the area of resection:

- Resection of the terminal ileum interferes with absorption of bile salts and vitamin B12. If less than 100 cm is removed, malabsorption of bile salts causes watery diarrhea. Treatment includes salt-binding resins (cholestyramine 2 to 4 g three times daily). If greater than 100 cm is removed, steatorrhea with resultant malabsorption of fat-soluble vitamins occurs. Additional treatment includes a low-fat diet, vitamins, and calcium supplements to prevent oxalate kidney stone.
- Resection of greater than 40% to 50% of small bowel results in weight loss, diarrhea, and electrolyte imbalance. If colon and 100 cm of proximal jejunum are retained, a low-fat, high-complex carbohydrate diet and electrolytes may maintain nutrition, but if the colon is removed, 200 cm of jejunum is required for adequate nutrition. Otherwise, parenteral nutrition is required, and this can lead to liver failure and death or liver/intestine transplantation.

Bariatric Surgery

Bariatric surgery is used to promote weight loss in the morbidly obese (100 lbs over normal weight or body mass index of 35 to 40). Surgery is done to restrict intake and/or prevent absorption of calories. Procedures are open surgical or laparoscopic and include:

- *Banding* places a band around the upper portion of the stomach, creating a small pouch with a small distal opening to slow emptying.
- *Sleeve gastrectomy* removes about two-thirds of stomach, and a distal part of the small intestine is attached directly to the remaining stomach, bypassing part of the small intestine to reduce absorption.
- *Roux-en-Y* uses staples and a vertical band to decrease the size of the stomach, creating a small pouch. Then a section of the small intestine is attached to the pouch, bypassing the first and second segments of the intestine to reduce absorption.
- *Gastric ballooning* places a balloon in the stomach and fills it with liquid to decrease stomach capacity. This is used primarily in Europe.

Gastrointestinal Surgeries

Cholecystectomy

Acute gallbladder disease is usually stabilized prior to surgery, except for acalculous cholecystitis or severe cholangitis, which may require emergency surgery. Traditional cholecystectomy requires an abdominal incision of about 5 to 8 inches and a hospital stay of a few days. There is usually significant discomfort as well as an extended recovery time. This procedure is usually reserved for those with adhesions or scarring from previous surgery. Cholecystectomy is now usually performed with laparoscopy with insufflation of carbon dioxide into the abdomen. Usually a number of small incisions are made to allow for passage of the laparoscope as well as instruments. Patients often are able to return home within a few hours of surgery, and discomfort is minimal. Complications of laparoscopy include damage to the bile duct, infection, and inadvertent injury to vessels or perforation of intestines.

Appendectomy

Appendectomy is usually required for acute appendicitis, which is inflammation of the appendix caused by luminal obstruction and pressure within the lumen; secretions build up and can eventually perforate the appendix. Appendicitis can occur in all ages, but infants and children younger than 2 years usually present with peritonitis or sepsis because of difficulty in early diagnosis. *Symptoms* include:

- acute abdominal pain, which may be epigastric, periumbilical, right lower quadrant, or right flank with rebound tenderness
- anorexia
- nausea and vomiting
- positive psoas and obturator signs
- fever may develop after 24 hours.

Diagnosis is based on clinical presentation, complete blood cell count (although leukocytosis may not be present), urinalysis, and imaging studies (such as x-rays, ultrasound, and CT). *Treatment* includes antibiotics, usually started on diagnosis, followed by surgical excision of the inflamed appendix. In rare cases of confined appendicitis (with mild symptoms), antibiotics alone may resolve the inflammation. Surgery is done under a general anesthesia through a small incision or with a minimally invasive laparoscopic approach.

Bowel Resection

Bowel resection because of malignancy, ischemia, trauma, or extensive disease may require a colostomy:

- *Descending/Sigmoid*: The descending or sigmoid colostomy is the most common type and creates a stoma from the end of the sigmoid (descending) colon, usually in the lower left abdomen.
- *Loop*: A loop colostomy creates one stoma with two openings, one for stool and the other for mucus, usually in the transverse colon. May have a supporting rod in place. This is a common procedure for short-term fecal diversion.
- *Transverse*: The transverse colostomy creates one or two stomas from the transverse colon, usually in the upper abdomen in the middle or on the right side.
- *End-loop*: Loop of intestine is brought to abdominal wall with both proximal and distal end stomas side by side. Often used as a temporary procedure for obstructed colon.
- *Hidden*: A loop of intestine is retained in subcutaneous fat and left for easy access in case a colostomy becomes necessary at a later date.

Ileostomy

End (standard, Brooke's): The end of the ileum is brought up through the abdominal wall to create a stoma, usually after the colon and rectum are surgically removed. If some colon and the rectum remain but are sutured closed and left below the surface, this type of ileostomy is a temporary procedure. The stoma is usually small and round and fairly easy to pouch.

Loop: A loop of the ileum is brought through the abdominal wall. A rod may be placed beneath the loop to keep it elevated above the skin. The loop is opened to allow for fecal drainage from the proximal portion of the loop and mucus from the distal portion. The loop is usually temporary, allowing the colon to heal, and this construction allows for easy closure of the ileostomy. Loop ileostomies tend to have larger misshapen stomas that are more difficult to pouch.

Colorectal Cancer

Reasons for colorectal surgery include:

- Prophylactic: To prevent cancer, often for precancerous polyps.
- Diagnostic: Biopsy to confirm diagnosis and determine type of cancer. Various surgical techniques may be used.
- Staging: To determine extent of malignant invasion. Surgical staging is more accurate than imaging or laboratory findings.

- Curative: Removal of tumor to effect a cure. It is considered the primary treatment but may be done in conjunction with chemotherapy or radiotherapy.
- Cytoreductive: Debulking removes all possible tumors without damaging organs or surrounding areas and may be done when it is impossible or too dangerous to remove entire tumor. It may be followed by chemotherapy or radiotherapy.
- Palliative: To alleviate symptoms or discomfort. Not curative.
- Supportive: To assist with other treatments. May include installation of catheter port into large vein for delivery of chemotherapy or blood testing.
- Restorative: To restore function, as when colostomy is removed and bowel reattached.

FECAL DIVERSION SURGERY

Indications for Fecal Diversion Surgery

Inflammatory bowel disease	*Crohn's disease* may affect any part of the GI system, especially the ileum. It may cause swelling and lesions that involve all layers of the intestinal wall. *Ulcerative colitis* causes inflammation and ulceration of the large intestine, but only in the top layer of the intestinal wall.
GI cancers	*Rectal or colon cancer* may metastasize or obstruct bowels. *Rectal obstruction* may result from metastasis of advanced pelvic cancer
GI and non-GI etiologies	*Diverticular disease* with complications may result in abscess, obstruction, fistula, or perforation of intestine. *Radiation enteritis* may cause malfunction from intestinal damage.
	Ischemic colitis most often of the left colon may cause irreversible damage. Infectious enteritis may be caused by bacteria, viruses, parasites, or fungi. Hospital stay and/or antibiotic use may lead to Clostridioides difficile infection, which may lead to severe complications. Intestinal obstruction, mechanical or non-mechanical, can lead to necrosis. GI trauma related to blunt or penetrating injuries may damage part of intestine.

HEPATIC DISEASES

CIRRHOSIS

Cirrhosis is a chronic hepatic disease in which healthy liver tissue is replaced the fibrotic tissue that impairs liver function. There are 3 types:

- *Alcoholic* (from chronic alcoholism) is the most common type and results in fibrosis about the portal areas. The liver cells become necrotic, replaced by fibrotic tissue, with areas of normal tissue projecting in between, giving the liver a hobnail appearance.
- *Postnecrotic* with broad bands of fibrotic tissue is the result of acute viral hepatitis.
- *Biliary*, the least common type, is caused by chronic biliary obstruction and cholangitis with resulting fibrotic tissue about the bile ducts.

Cirrhosis may be either compensated or decompensated.

- *Compensated* cirrhosis usually involves nonspecific symptoms, such as intermittent fever, epistaxis, ankle edema, indigestion, abdominal pain, and palmar erythema. Hepatomegaly and splenomegaly may also be present.
- *Decompensated cirrhosis* occurs when the liver can no longer adequately synthesize proteins, clotting factors, and other substances so that portal hypertension occurs. *Symptoms* include:
- hepatomegaly, portal obstruction resulting in jaundice and ascites
- chronic elevated temperature; purpura resulting from thrombocytopenia, with bruising and epistaxis.
- bacterial peritonitis may develop with ascites

- esophageal varices; edema of extremities and presacral area resulting from reduced albumin in the plasma
- vitamin deficiency from interference with formation, use, and storage of vitamins, such as A, C, and K
- anemia from chronic gastritis and decreased dietary intake, anemia
- hepatic encephalopathy with alterations in mentation
- Hypotension; atrophy of gonads.

Treatment varies according to the symptoms and is supportive rather than curative as the fibrotic changes in the liver cannot be reversed: dietary supplements and vitamins; diuretics (potassium sparing), such as spironolactone and triamterene, to decrease ascites; colchicine to reduce fibrotic changes; and liver transplant, the definitive treatment

Hepatitis A and B

Hepatitis A virus (HAV), an RNA picornavirus that replicates in the liver, is secreted into the gallbladder and enters the intestines. The virus triggers an antibody-mediated immune response with immunoglobulin M (IgM) that confers immunity, so reinfection and chronic infection does not occur. HAV infection is often asymptomatic in children, but adults may develop jaundice, general malaise, pain in the abdomen, nausea, and diarrhea. The virus is transmitted by the oral-fecal route, often from contamination on the hands or through sexual contact. On rare occasions, HAV has been transmitted in blood transfusions.

Hepatitis B virus (HBV) is a DNA virus of the family *Hepadnaviridae*. It is transmitted through contact with blood either directly, or through sexual contact or sharing needles. The DNA genome enters the host cell nucleus, copies, and replicates. The cell-mediated immune response that destroys the virus also causes damage to hepatic cells, resulting in acute hepatitis. Chronic infection occurs in 90% of infants but 6% of those older than 5 years old, with 15% to 25% of those with chronic infection developing liver cancer.

Hepatitis C Virus

Hepatitis C virus (HCV) is a single-strand RNA *Flaviviridae* virus that binds to receptors on hepatic cells and enters to begin replicating. HCV readily mutates, which helps it to evade the host's immune response. There are 6 genotypes and several subtypes of HCV with some types more virulent and resistive to treatment than others. There is no vaccine. HCV is transmitted directly through blood or items such as shared needles that are contaminated with blood. It can be spread by sexual contact. Prior to 1992, the blood supply was contaminated with HCV as were clotting factors made before 1987. HCV causes an acute infection (first 6 months), but 55% to 85% develop chronic infection with 70% of those developing chronic liver disease. HCV is the primary reason for liver transplants.

Hepatic Failure

Hepatic failure occurs when the liver is no longer able to function. The liver receives oxygenated blood from the right and left hepatic arteries and blood rich in nutrients from the intestinal tract through the portal vein. Portal venous blood is normally filtered in the liver, and pathogens and nutrients are absorbed and metabolized by hepatocytes. Nutrients are stored in the liver or excreted into the hepatic veins and inferior vena cava. With liver failure, this process is impaired by *portal hypertension*.

The portal vein that feeds the liver becomes obstructed, reducing blood flow and increasing blood pressure in the portal venous system, which is already compressed by cirrhotic changes. The liver cannot filter blood adequately, and the increased pressure creates collateral blood vessels that bypass the obstruction, returning unfiltered blood to the systemic circulation as a result. Collateral vessels cause varices to form in the esophagus or other areas. Increased aldosterone causes sodium and fluid retention. Plasma albumin decreases, causing fluid to leak from the vascular system and resulting in ascites.

Conditions other than portal hypertension that are part of the syndrome of liver failure:

- *Hepatorenal syndrome* results in marked decrease in renal blood flow with resultant increase in azotemia (nitrogenous substances). Sodium levels fall and potassium increases, and there are multiple abnormalities in blood chemistries and clotting times. Hepatorenal syndrome is often related to hepatic encephalopathy.
- *Hepatic encephalopathy* occurs when ammonia crosses the blood-brain barrier and is absorbed by brain tissue. Normally, when protein is digested in the intestines, the ammonia that is produced as a byproduct is filtered by the liver and metabolized to form urea. When blood flow from the portal system is restricted, the serum ammonia level increases. Ammonia causes increasing confusion, stupor, and coma with marked changes in electroencephalogram (EEG).

FULMINANT HEPATITIS/LIVER FAILURE

Fulminant hepatitis/liver failure is a severe life-threatening acute liver infection. It may be triggered by in hepatitis or other viruses, toxins (carbon tetrachloride), Wilson disease, and drugs, most commonly acetaminophen, a drug frequently used by teenagers for suicide attempts. Fulminant hepatitis has a very rapid onset with jaundice, hepatic necrosis, hepatic encephalopathy, coma, and death often within days. However, in some cases, liver failure may be delayed. It is classified according to the time of liver failure:

- Hyperacute: 0 to 7 days
- Acute: 8 to 28 days
- Subacute: 28 to 72 days.

Symptoms vary but anorexia is common. Intracranial pressure increases as encephalopathy and cerebral edema occur, and this can result in brainstem compression. As the condition worsens, coagulopathies may cause GI bleeding. Renal failure occurs with electrolyte imbalances. Sepsis often leads to multiorgan failure, and death occurs in 80% of patients.

ACUTE ABDOMINAL TRAUMA

Acute abdominal trauma may be blunt or penetrating:

- *Blunt injuries* from motor vehicle accident (MVA), sports injuries, falls, and assaults are common causes of abdominal injury and comprise crush (compression), shear (tearing), and burst (sudden increased pressure). MVA often results in liver injury in the passenger with impact on that side and spleen injury in the driver with impact on the driver's side. Other injuries from blunt trauma include damage to the diaphragm, retroperitoneal hematomas, and intestinal injuries, including perforation.
- *Penetrating wounds,* on the other hand, are almost always related to gunshot wounds (high energy) or knife assaults (low energy). Gunshot wounds tend to cause more extensive damage than stab wounds, especially to the colon, liver, spleen and diaphragm. Interior injury may be extensive because the bullet damages tissue and may ricochet off of bone. Hemorrhage and peritonitis are common complications.

SPLENIC INJURY

The spleen is the most frequently injured solid organ in blunt trauma. Injuries to the spleen are the most common because it is not well protected by the rib cage and is very vascular. *Symptoms* may be very nonspecific. Kehr sign (radiating pain in left shoulder) indicates intra-abdominal bleeding and Cullen sign (ecchymosis around umbilicus) indicates hemorrhage from ruptured spleen. Some may have right upper abdominal pain although diffuse abdominal pain often occurs with blood loss, associated with hypotension. Splenic injuries are classified according to the degree of injury:

1. Tear in splenic capsules or hematoma.
2. Laceration of parenchyma (less than 3 cm).

3. Laceration of parenchyma (greater than 3 cm).
4. Multiple lacerations of parenchyma or burst-type injury.

Treatment may be supportive if injury is not severe; otherwise, suturing of spleen may be needed. Because there is a risk of infection with splenectomy, every effort (bed rest, transfusion, reduced activity for at least 8 weeks) is done to avoid surgery because the spleen will often heal spontaneously.

Hepatic Injuries

Hepatic injury is the most common cause of death (mortality rates of 8% to 25%) from abdominal trauma and is often associated with multiple organ damage, so symptoms may be nonspecific. Automobile accidents cause most blunt trauma. Elevation in liver transaminase levels indicates damage that may require CT examination with double contrast. Liver injuries are classified according to the degree of injury:

I. Tears in capsule with hematoma.
II. Laceration(s) of parenchyma (1 to 3 cm).
III. Laceration(s) of parenchyma (greater than 3 cm).
IV. Destruction of 25% to 75% of lobe from burst injury.
V. Destruction of more than 75% of lobe from burst injury.
VI. Avulsion [tearing away].

Hemodynamically stable patients are managed medically, but surgical repair may be necessary if the patient is unstable or bleeding. Hemorrhage is common complication of hepatic injury and may require ligation of hepatic arteries or veins. *Treatment* often includes IV fluids for fluid volume deficit, as well as blood products (plasma, platelets) for coagulopathies.

Gastric and Intestinal Injuries

Gastric injuries may result in perforation, primarily at the greater curvature. The risk increases if the person is injured with a full stomach after eating a meal and suffers blunt or penetrating force to the abdomen. Perforation results in severe pain, rigid abdomen, and bloody nasogastric drainage with peritonitis developing within hours, so early diagnosis and surgical repair must be done. Intestinal injuries may occur from blunt or penetrating trauma. Indications of rupture often appear 24 to 48 hours when the person presents with symptoms of peritonitis resulting from leakage of intestinal contents into the peritoneum. Symptoms may include distention, abdominal pain, absent bowel sounds, leukocytosis, fever, dyspnea, nausea, and vomiting. Sepsis and abscess or fistula formation can occur. Treatment includes prompt antibiotic therapy and surgical repair with peritoneal lavage. The abdominal wound may be left open to heal by secondary intention.

Compartment Syndrome

Abdominal trauma with pronounced shock increases risk of compartment syndrome for a number of reasons:

- edema of the intestines because of trauma and surgical manipulation
- capillary leakage
- hemorrhage (retroperitoneal)
- abdominal packing left in place to control bleeding
- IV crystalloid administration.

Pressure within the abdomen may begin to rise rapidly if the abdomen is closed, resulting in decreased cardiac output from pressure on the vena cava, increased airway pressures and acute respiratory distress syndrome, decreased urinary output with decrease in renal blood flow and glomerular filtration, increased central venous pressure resulting in increased intracranial pressure and cerebral edema. *Diagnosis* is by measurement of intra-abdominal pressure (greater than 25 cm H_2O) by Foley catheter or NG tube with pressure transducer or water-column manometry. If risk for compartment syndrome exists, the wound should not be closed. Sudden release of pressure and reperfusion may cause acidosis, vasodilation, and cardiac arrest, so the patient should be given crystalloid solutions before decompression.

Renal

Acute and Chronic Renal Failure

Acute Tubular Necrosis

Acute tubular necrosis (ATN) occurs when a hypoxic condition causes renal ischemia that damages tubular cells of the glomeruli so they are unable to adequately filter the urine, leading to acute renal failure. Causes include hypotension, hyperbilirubinemia, sepsis, surgery (especially cardiac or vascular), and birth complications. ATN may result from nephrotoxic injury related to obstruction or drugs, such as chemotherapy, acyclovir, and antibiotics, such as sulfonamides and streptomycin.

Symptoms may be nonspecific initially and include life-threatening complications: Lethargy, nausea and vomiting, hypovolemia with low cardiac output and generalized vasodilation, fluid and electrolyte imbalance leading to hypertension, CNS abnormalities, metabolic acidosis, arrhythmias, edema, and congestive heart failure,uremia leading to destruction of platelets and bleeding, neurological deficits, and disseminated intravascular coagulopathy (DIC),infections can include pericarditis and sepsis.

Treatment includes:

- identifying and treating underlying cause
- supportive care, loop diuretics (in some cases), such as Lasix®.
- antibiotics for infection, discontinuation of nephrotoxic agents
- kidney dialysis.

Chronic Renal Failure

Renal failure occurs when the kidneys are unable to filter and excrete wastes, concentrate urine, and maintain electrolyte balance because of hypoxic conditions, kidney disease, or obstruction in the urinary tract. It results first in azotemia (increase in nitrogenous waste in the blood) and then in uremia (nitrogenous wastes cause toxic symptoms. When more than 50% of the functional renal capacity is destroyed, the kidneys can no longer carry out necessary functions and progressive deterioration (end-stage renal disease) begins over months or years.

- *Symptoms* are often nonspecific in the beginning with loss of appetite and energy: weight loss, headaches, muscle cramping, general malaise, increased bruising and dry or itching skin, increased BUN and creatinine, sodium and fluid retention with edema, Hyperkalemia, metabolic acidosis, calcium and phosphorus depletion, resulting in altered bone metabolism, pain, and retarded growth, anemia with decreased production on RBCs, increased risk of infection, uremic syndrome.
- *Treatment:* supportive/symptomatic therapy, dialysis and transplantation.
- *Renal dialysis* is used primarily for those who have progressed from renal insufficiency to uremia with end-stage renal disease (ESRD). It may also be used temporarily for acute conditions. Patients can be maintained on dialysis, but there are many complications associated with dialysis so many patients are considered for renal transplantation. There are a number of different approaches to dialysis:
- *Peritoneal dialysis*: an indwelling catheter is inserted surgically into the peritoneal cavity with a subcutaneous tunnel and a Dacron cuff to prevent infection. Sterile dialysate solution is slowly instilled through gravity, remains for a prescribed length of time, and is then drained and discarded. In *continuous ambulatory peritoneal dialysis*, a series of exchange cycles are repeated 24 hours a day. In *continuous cyclic peritoneal dialysis*, a prolonged period of retaining fluid occurs during the day with drainage at night. Peritoneal dialysis may be used for those who want to be more independent, do not live near a dialysis center, or want fewer dietary restrictions.

Cerebral Hypoxia

Cerebral hypoxia (hypoxic encephalopathy) occurs when the oxygen supply to the brain is decreased. If hypoxia is mild, the brain compensates by increasing cerebral blood flow, but it can only double in volume and cannot compensate for severe hypoxic conditions. Hypoxia may be the result of insufficient oxygen in the environment, inadequate exchange at the alveolar level of the lungs, or inadequate circulation to the brain. Brain cells may begin dying within 5 minutes if deprived of adequate oxygenation, so any condition or trauma that interferes with oxygenation can result in brain damage:

- near-drowning
- asphyxia
- cardiac arrest
- high-altitude sickness
- carbon monoxide
- diseases that interfere with respiration, such as myasthenia gravis and amyotrophic lateral sclerosis
- anesthesia complications.

Symptoms include increasing neurological deficits, depending upon the degree and area of damage, with changes in mentation that range from confusion to coma. Prompt identification of the cause and increase in perfusion to the brain is critical for survival.

Hemodialysis

Hemodialysis, the most common type of dialysis, is used for both short-term dialysis and long-term for those with ESRD. Treatments are usually done 3 times weekly for 3 to 4 hours or short daily dialysis with treatment either during the night or in short daily periods. Hemodialysis is often done for those who cannot manage peritoneal dialysis or who live near a dialysis center, but it does interfere with work or school attendance and requires strict dietary and fluid restrictions between treatments. Short daily dialysis allows more independence, and increased costs may be offset by lower morbidity. A vascular access device, such as a catheter, fistula, or graft, must be established for hemodialysis, and heparin is used to prevent clotting. With hemodialysis, blood is circulated outside of the body through a dialyzer (a synthetic semipermeable membrane), which filters the blood. There are many different types of dialyzers. High-flux dialyzers use a highly permeable membrane that shortens the duration of treatment and decreases the need for heparin.

Continuous Renal Replacement Therapy

Continuous renal replacement therapy (CCRT) circulates the blood by hydrostatic pressure through a semipermeable membrane. It is used in acute/critical care and can be instituted quickly:

- *Continuous arteriovenous hemofiltration* (CAVH) circulates blood from an artery (usually the femoral) to a hemofilter using only arterial pressure and not a blood pump. The filtered blood is then returned to the patient's venous system, often with added fluids to offset those lost. Only the fluid in filtered.
- *Continuous arteriovenous hemodialysis* (CAVHD) is similar to CAVH except that dialysate circulates on one side of the semipermeable membrane to increase clearance of urea.
- *Continuous venovenous hemofiltration* (CVVH) pumps blood through a double-lumen venous catheter to a hemofilter, which returns the blood to the patient in the same catheter. It provides continuous slow removal of fluid, is better tolerated with unstable patients, and does not require arterial access.
- *Continuous venovenous hemodialysis* is similar to CVVH but uses a dialysate to increase clearance of uremic toxins.

Complications Associated with Dialysis

There are many **complications** associated with dialysis, especially when used for long-term treatment:

- ***Hemodialysis***: Long-term use promotes atherosclerosis and cardiovascular disease. Anemia and fatigue are common, as are infections related to access devices or contamination of equipment. Some patients experience hypotension and muscle cramping during treatment. Dysrhythmias may occur. Some may exhibit dialysis disequilibrium from cerebral fluid shifts, causing headaches, nausea and vomiting, and alterations of consciousness.

- ***Peritoneal dialysis***: Most complications are minor, but it can lead to peritonitis, which requires removal of the catheter if antibiotic therapy is not successful in clearing the infection within 4 days. There may be leakage of the dialysate around the catheter. Bleeding may occur, especially in women who are menstruating as blood is pulled from the uterus through the fallopian tubes. Abdominal hernias may occur with long use. Some may have anorexia from feeling of fullness or sweet taste in mouth from absorption of glucose.

REGULATORY FUNCTIONS

The kidneys produce urine, but that is a byproduct of the primary regulatory functions:

- *Waste excretion* of metabolic products such as urea, creatinine, phosphates, sulfates, uric acid, and drug metabolites prevents toxic reactions.
- *Electrolyte excretion* should equal the amount ingested in normal functioning. Most fluid and sodium filtered through the glomeruli are reabsorbed into the blood before the urine leaves the body. The amount of sodium reabsorbed controls the amount of fluid reabsorbed. If more sodium is excreted than ingested, it results in dehydration. If less sodium is excreted than ingested, it results in fluid retention. Aldosterone, produced in the renal cortex, controls both the excretion of sodium and potassium. Increased levels cause reabsorption of sodium and excretion of potassium.
- *Acid excretion* rids the body of the products of protein catabolism (breakdown) either directly in the urine or bound to phosphate and ammonia ions.

Regulatory functions, including fluid and electrolyte balance, of the kidneys include:

Water excretion balances intake with output so increased intake results in a large output and vice versa.

- *Osmolality* (the number of electrolytes and other molecules per kg water) measures the concentration or dilution. With dehydration, osmolality increases; with fluid retention, osmolality decreases. With kidney disease, urine is dilute and the osmolality is fixed.
- *Specific gravity* compares the weight of urine (weight of particles) to distilled water (1.000). Normal urine is 1.010 to 1.025 with normal intake. High intake lowers the specific gravity and low intake raises it. In kidney disease, it often does not vary.
- *Antidiuretic hormone* (ADH/vasopressin) regulates the excretion of water and urine concentration in the renal tubule by varying water reabsorption. When fluid intake decreases, blood osmolality rises and this stimulates release of ADH, which increases reabsorption of fluid to return osmolality to normal levels.

Regulatory functions of the kidneys include:

- *Blood pressure* is regulated by special vessels (vasa recta) that stimulate renin production with hypotension. Renin converts angiotensinogen to angiotensin II, a powerful vasoconstrictor, and the vasoconstriction increases blood pressure. Renin production stops when blood pressure rises. Failure of this system results in hypertension.
- *Renal clearance* is the ability of kidney to filter solutes, such as creatinine. Creatinine clearance is used to evaluate renal function; clearance decreases when renal function decreases.
- *Red blood cell production* is stimulated by the kidney's production of erythropoietin in the presence of decreased oxygen tension, increasing red blood cells to increase the availability of hemoglobin to carry oxygen.
- *Vitamin D synthesis* is completed in the kidneys. Vitamin D is necessary for the maintenance of normal calcium values.
- *Secretion of prostaglandin* provides vasodilation to maintain renal blood flow.

Polycystic Kidney Disease

Polycystic kidney disease (PKD) is caused by renal cysts that develop from nephrons and can cause gross enlargement of kidneys. Cysts may be single or multiple (polycystic) and may involve one or both kidneys. There are 2 types of congenital PKD:

- *Autosomal dominant* is the most common (90%), but symptoms are usually delayed until adulthood although they can occur in infancy. Cysts may develop in any part of the nephron. It may progress to ESRD over time. Cysts may also form in the liver and pancreas. It is associated with cerebral artery aneurysms.
- *Autosomal recessive* is rarer and symptoms arise much earlier, sometimes in the fetus. It is always bilateral with enlarged kidneys.

Both types of PKD often manifest with abdominal mass (sometimes bilateral flank), oliguria, acute renal failure, Potter facies (related to oligohydramnios), hypoplastic lungs, respiratory distress, and hypertension.

Treatment cannot cure but can delay effects:

- antihypertensives
- antibiotics for infections
- analgesia
- growth hormone (autosomal recessive)
- long-term: dialysis and transplantation.

Hydronephrosis

Hydronephrosis is a symptom of a disease involving swelling of the kidney pelvises and calyces because of an obstruction that causes urine to be retained in the kidney. In chronic conditions, symptoms may be delayed until severe kidney damage has occurred. Over time, the kidney begins to atrophy. The primary condition conditions that predispose to hydronephrosis include:

- vesicoureteral reflux
- obstruction at the ureteropelvic junction
- renal edema (nonobstructive).

Any condition that impairs drainage of the ureters can cause backup of the urine. *Symptoms* vary widely depending upon cause and whether the condition is acute or chronic. Acute episodes are usually characterized by flank pain, abnormal creatinine and electrolyte levels, and increased pH. The enlarged kidney may be palpable as a soft mass. *Treatment* requires identifying the cause of obstruction and correcting it to ensure adequate drainage. A nephrostomy tube, ureteral stent, or pyeloplasty may be done surgically in some cases. A urinary catheter may be inserted if there is outflow obstruction from the bladder.

Renal and Ureteral Calculi

Renal and urinary calculi occur frequently, more commonly in males, and can relate to diseases (hyperparathyroidism, renal tubular acidosis, gout) and lifestyle factors, such as sedentary work. Additionally, some medications can precipitate calculi. Calculi can form at any age, most composed of calcium, and can range in size from very tiny to greater than 6 mm. Those less than 4 mm can usually pass in the urine easily. *Symptoms* occur with obstruction and are usually of sudden onset and acute:

- severe flank pain radiating to abdomen and ipsilateral testicle or labium majorum, abdominal or pelvic pain (young children)
- nausea and vomiting
- diaphoresis
- hematuria.

Diagnostic studies include clinical findings, uric acid (UA), pregnancy test to rule out ectopic pregnancy, BUN and creatinine if indicated, ultrasound (for pregnant women and children), IV urography. Helical CT (noncontrast) is diagnostic.

Treatments include:

- analgesia: opiates and NSAIDs
- instructions and equipment for straining urine
- antibiotics if concurrent infection
- referral to urologist for large calculi.

PYELONEPHRITIS

Pyelonephritis is a potentially organ-damaging bacterial infection of the parenchyma of the kidney. Pyelonephritis can result in abscess formation, sepsis, and kidney failure. Pyelonephritis is especially dangerous for those who are immunocompromised, pregnant, or diabetic. Most infections are caused by *Escherichia coli.*

Symptoms vary widely but can include:

- dysuria and frequency, hematuria, flank and/or low back pain
- fever and chills
- costovertebral angle tenderness
- change in feeding habits (infants)
- change in mental status (geriatric)

Younger women often exhibit symptoms more associated with lower urinary infection, so the condition may be overlooked. Patients may require hospitalization or careful follow-up. *Diagnostic* studies include urinalysis, and blood and urine cultures. *Treatments* include:

- analgesia
- antipyretics
- IV fluids
- antibiotics are started initially but may be changed based on cultures:
    - IV ceftriaxone with fluoroquinolone orally for 14 days
    - fluoroquinolone orally for 14 days.

CYSTITIS

Urinary infections, cystitis, are common and often chronic, low-grade kidney infections develop over time, so observing for *symptoms* of urinary infections and treating promptly are very important.

Changes in character of urine:

- *Appearance*: The urine may become cloudy from mucus or purulent material. Hematuria may be present.
- *Color*: Urine usually becomes concentrated and may be dark yellow/orange or brownish in color.
- *Odor:* Urine may have a very strong or foul odor.
- *Output*: Urinary output may decrease markedly.
- Pain**:** There may be lower back or flank pain from inflammation of the kidneys.

Systemic: Fever, chills, headache, and general malaise often accompany urine infections. Some people suffer lack of appetite as well as nausea and vomiting. Fever usually indicates that the infection has affected the kidneys. Children may develop incontinence or loose stools and cry excessively.

Treatment: Increased fluid intake and antibiotics.

Arterial Blood Gases (ABGs)

Arterial blood gases (ABGs) are monitored to assess effectiveness of oxygenation, ventilation, and acid-base status, and to determine oxygen flow rates. Partial pressure of a gas is that exerted by each gas in a mixture of gases, proportional to its concentration, based on total atmospheric pressure of 760 mm Hg at sea level. Normal values include:

- Acidity/Alkalinity (pH): 7.35 to 7.45.
- Partial pressure of carbon dioxide ($PaCO_2$): 35 to 45 mm Hg.
- Partial pressure of oxygen (PaO_2): at least 80 mm Hg.
- Bicarbonate concentration (HCO_3): 22 to 26 mEq/L.
- Oxygen saturation (SaO_2): at least 95%.

The relationship between these elements, particularly the $PaCO_2$ and the PaO_2, indicates respiratory status. For example, $PaCO_2$ greater than 55 and the PaO_2 less than 60 in a patient previously in good health indicates respiratory failure. There are many issues to consider. Ventilator management may require a higher $PaCO_2$ to prevent barotrauma and a lower PaO_2 to reduce oxygen toxicity.

Review Video: Blood Gases
Visit mometrix.com/academy and enter code: 611909

Nutritional Status

Total protein levels can be influenced by many factors, including stress and infection, but it may be monitored as part of an overall nutritional assessment. Protein is critical for wound healing, and because metabolic rate increases in response to a wound, protein needs increase:

- Normal values: 0.8 g of protein per kg per body weight per day.
- Diet requirements for wound healing: 1.25 to 1.5 g/kg per day.

Albumin is a protein that is produced by the liver and is a necessary component for cells and tissues. Levels decrease with renal disease, malnutrition, and severe burns. Albumin levels are the most common screening to determine protein levels. Albumin has a half-life of 18 to 20 days, so it is sensitive to long-term protein deficiencies more than short-term.

- Normal values: 3.5 to 5.5 g/dL
- Mild deficiency: 3 to 3.5 g/dL
- Moderate deficiency: 2.5 to 3 g/dL
- Severe deficiency: less than 2.5 g/dL.

Levels below 3.2 correlate with increased morbidity and death. Dehydration (poor intake, diarrhea, or vomiting) elevates levels, so adequate hydration is important to ensure meaningful results.

Nutritional Status (Prealbumin)

Prealbumin (transthyretin) is most commonly monitored for acute changes in nutritional status because it has a half-life of only 2 to 3 days. Prealbumin is a protein produced in the liver, so it is often decreased with liver disease. Oral contraceptives and estrogen can also decrease levels. Levels may rise with Hodgkin's disease or the use of steroids or NSAIDs. Prealbumin is necessary for transportation of both thyroxine and vitamin A throughout the body, so if levels fall, both thyroxine and vitamin A utilization are also affected.

- Normal values: 16 to 40 mg/dL
- Mild deficiency: 10 to 15 mg/dL

- Moderate deficiency: 5 to 9 mg/dL
- Severe deficiency: less than 5 mg/dL

Prealbumin is a good measurement because it quickly decreases when nutrition is inadequate and rises quickly in response to increased protein intake. Protein intake must be adequate to maintain levels of prealbumin. Death rates increase with any decrease in prealbumin levels.

Nutritional Status (Transferrin)

Transferrin, which transports about one-third of the body's iron, is a protein produced by the liver. It transports iron from the intestines to the bone marrow where it is used to produce hemoglobin. The half-life of transferrin is about 8 to 10 days. It is sometimes used as a measure of nutritional status; however, transferrin levels are sensitive to many different things. Levels rapidly decrease with protein malnutrition.

Liver disease and anemia can also depress levels, but a decrease in iron, commonly found with inadequate protein, stimulates the liver to produce more transferrin, which increases levels but also decreases production of albumin and prealbumin. Levels may also increase with pregnancy, use of oral contraceptives, and polycythemia. Thus, transferrin levels alone are not always reliable measurements of nutritional status:

- Normal values: 200 to 400 mg/dL
- Mild deficiency: 150 to 200 mg/dL
- Moderate deficiency: 100 to 150 mg/dL
- Severe deficiency: less than 100 mg/dL.

Nutritional Status, Immune Disorders

The immune system responds quickly to changes in protein intake because proteins are critical to antibody and lymphocyte production. T lymphocytes develop in the thymus gland and are a part of the cell-mediated immune response. B-lymphocytes develop in the bone marrow and are part of the humoral (antibody-mediated) immune response. Total lymphocyte count (TLC) can reflect changes in nutritional status because a decrease in protein causes decreased immunity. Lymphocytes are expressed on a differential as a percentage of the white blood cell count. The TLC is calculated by multiplying the percentage by the total white blood cell count and then dividing by 100.

- Normal values: 2,000 cells/mm^3
- Mild deficiency: 1,500 to 1,800 cells/mm^3
- Moderate deficiency: 900 to 1,500 cells/mm^3
- Severe deficiency: less than 900 cells/mm^3.

While low levels may be indicative of malnutrition, levels are also depressed with stress, autoimmune diseases, chemotherapy, infection, and HIV.

Distributive Shock

Distributive shock occurs with adequate blood volume but inadequate intravascular volume because of arterial/venous dilation that results in decreased vascular tone and hypoperfusion of internal organs. Cardiac output may be normal or blood may pool, decreasing cardiac output. Distributive shock may result from anaphylactic shock, septic shock, neurogenic shock, and drug ingestions.

Symptoms: hypotension (systolic less than 90 mm Hg or mean arterial blood pressure less than 60 mm Hg), tachypnea, tachycardia (greater than 90 beats per minute; may be lower if patient receiving beta-blockers), skin initially warm, later hypoperfused, hyper- or hypothermia (more than 38ºC or less than 36ºC), hypoxemia, alterations in mentation, increased urinary output, symptoms related to underlying cause.

Diagnostic procedures are similar to those for septic and anaphylactic shock. *Treatment* includes treating underlying cause and stabilizing hemodynamics: septic shock or anaphylactic therapy and monitoring as indicated, oxygen with endotracheal intubation if necessary, rapid fluid administration at 0.25 to 0.5 L of NS or isotonic crystalloid every 5 to 10 minutes as needed to 2 to 3 L. (Children: 5 to 10 mL/kg to 30 mL/kg maximum) inotropes (dopamine, dobutamine, norepinephrine) if necessary,

Anaphylaxis Syndrome

Anaphylaxis syndrome is a sudden acute systemic immunoglobulin E (IgE) or non-IgE inflammatory response affecting the cardiopulmonary and other systems.

- *IgE-mediated response* (anaphylactic shock) is an antibody-antigen reaction against an allergen, such as milk, peanuts, latex, insect bites, or fish. This is the most common type.
- *Non-IgE–mediated response* (anaphylactoid reaction) is a systemic reaction to infection, exercise, radiocontrast material, or other triggers. While the response is almost identical to the other type, it does not involve IgE.

Typically, with IgE-mediated response, an antigen triggers release of substances, such as histamine and prostaglandins, which affect the skin, cardiopulmonary, and GI systems. Histamine causes initial erythema and edema by inducing vasodilation. Each time the person has contact with the antigen, more antibodies form in response, so allergic reactions worsen with each contact. In some cases, initial reactions may be mild, but subsequent contact can cause a severe life-threatening response.

Anaphylaxis Syndrome

Anaphylaxis syndrome may present with a few symptoms or a wide range that encompasses cardiopulmonary, dermatological, and GI responses.

Symptoms may recur after the initial treatment (biphasic anaphylaxis) so careful monitoring is essential:

- sudden onset of weakness, dizziness, confusion
- severe generalized edema and angioedema; lips and tongue may swell, urticaria, increased permeability of vascular system and loss of vascular tone, severe hypotension leading to shock
- laryngospasm/bronchospasm with obstruction of airway causing dyspnea and wheezing, nausea, vomiting, and diarrhea
- seizures, coma, and death.

Treatment includes:

- Establish patent airway and intubated if necessary for ventilation.
- provide oxygen at 100% high flow, monitor vital signs (VS)
- administer epinephrine (EpiPen or 1:1000 solution [0.1 mg/kg/wt])
- albuterol 2.5 mg per nebulizer for bronchospasm
- IV fluids to provide bolus of fluids for hypotension
- diphenhydramine 1.0 mg/kg/wt (to 25 mg) if shock persists
- methylprednisolone 2.0 mg/kg/wt is no response to other drugs.

Electrolyte Imbalances and Fluid Management

Fluid Balance

Body fluid is primarily intracellular fluid (ICF) or extracellular space (ECF). By 3 years of age, the fluid balance has stabilized and remains throughout adulthood:

- ECF: 20% to 30% (intrastitial fluid, plasma, transcellular fluid)
- ICF: 40% to 50% (fluid within the cells).

The fluid compartments are separated by semipermeable membranes that allow fluid and solutes (electrolytes and other substances) to move by osmosis. Fluid also moves through diffusion, filtration, and active transport. In fluid volume deficit, fluid is out of balance and ECF is depleted; an overload occurs with increased concentration of sodium and retention of fluid. Signs of fluid deficit include:

- thirsty, restless to lethargic
- increasing pulse rate, tachycardia
- fontanels depressed (infants)
- decreased urinary output
- normal BP progressing to hypotension
- dry mucous membranes

3% to 10% decrease in body weight.

Electrolyte Imbalances (Sodium)

Sodium (Na) regulates fluid volume, osmolality, acid-base balance, and activity in the muscles, nerves, and myocardium. It is the primary cation (positive ion) in ECF, necessary to maintain ECF levels that are needed for tissue perfusion:

- Normal value: 135 to 145 mEq/L.
- Hyponatremia: less than 135 mEq/L.
- Hypernatremia: greater than 145 mEq/L.

Hyponatremia may result from inadequate sodium intake or excess loss, through diarrhea, vomiting, or NG suctioning. It can occur as the result of illness, such as severe burns, fever, SIADH, and ketoacidosis. Symptoms vary:

- irritability to lethargy and alterations in consciousness
- cerebral edema with seizures and coma
- dyspnea to respiratory failure.
- *Treatment: A*nd treat underlying cause and provide Na replacement.

Hypernatremia may result from renal disease, diabetes insipidus, and fluid depletion. Symptoms include irritability to lethargy to confusion to coma, seizures, flushing, muscle weakness and spasms, and thirst. Treatment includes identifying and treating underlying cause, monitoring Na levels carefully, and IV fluid replacement.

Electrolyte Imbalances (Potassium Depletion)

Potassium (K) is the primary electrolyte in ICF with about 98% inside cells and only 2% in ECF, although this small amount is important for neuromuscular activity. K influences activity of the skeletal and cardiac muscles. K level is dependent upon adequate renal functioning because 80% is excreted through the kidneys and 20% through the bowels and sweat:

- Normal values: 3.5 to 5.5 mEq/L
- Hypokalemia: less than 3.5 mEq/L.

Hypokalemia is caused by loss of K through diarrhea, vomiting, gastric suction, diuresis, alkalosis, decreased K intake with starvation, and nephritis. *Symptoms* include:

- lethargy and weakness
- nausea and vomiting
- paresthesias
- dysrhythmias with ECG abnormalities: premature ventricular complexes (PVCs), flattened T waves

- muscle cramps with hyporeflexia
- hypotension
- tetany.

Treatment: Identify and treat underlying cause and replace K.

Electrolyte Imbalances (Potassium Excess)

Hyperkalemia is caused by renal disease, adrenal insufficiency, metabolic acidosis, severe dehydration, burns, hemolysis, and trauma. It rarely occurs without renal disease but may be induced by treatment (such as nsaids and potassium-sparing diuretics). Untreated renal failure results in reduced excretion. Those with Addison's disease and deficient adrenal hormones suffer sodium loss that results in potassium retention:

- hyperkalemia: greater than 5.5 mEq/L.

The primary symptoms relates to the effect on the cardiac muscle:

- ventricular arrhythmias with increasing changes in EKC leading to cardiac and respiratory arrest
- weakness with ascending paralysis and hyperreflexia
- diarrhea
- increasing confusion.

Treatment includes identifying underlying cause and discontinuing sources of increased K:

- calcium gluconate to decrease cardiac effects
- sodium bicarbonate shifts K into the cells temporarily
- insulin and hypertonic dextrose shift K into the cells temporarily
- cation exchange resin (sodium polystyrene) to decrease K
- peritoneal dialysis or hemodialysis.

Electrolyte Imbalances (Calcium)

More than 99% of **calcium (Ca)** is in the skeletal system with 1% in serum, but it is important for transmitting nerve impulses and regulating muscle contraction and relaxation, including the myocardium. Calcium activates enzymes that stimulate chemical reactions and has a role in coagulation of blood:

- Normal values: 1.15 to 1.34 mg/dL
- Hypocalcemia: less than 1.15 mg/dL
- Hypercalcemia: more than 1.34 mg/dL.

Hypocalcemia may be caused by hypoparathyroidism and occurs after thyroid and parathyroid surgery, pancreatitis, renal failure, inadequate vitamin D, alkalosis, magnesium deficiency and low serum albumin. *Symptoms* include:

- tetany, tingling, seizures, altered mental status
- ventricular tachycardia.

Treatment: calcium replacement and vitamin D.

Hypercalcemia may be caused by acidosis, kidney disease, hyperparathyroidism, prolonged immobilization, and malignancies. Crisis carries a 50% mortality rate. Symptoms include:

- increasing muscle weakness with hypotonicity
- anorexia, nausea and vomiting

- constipation
- bradycardia and cardiac arrest

Treatment: Identify and treat underlying cause, loop diuretics, and IV fluids.

Electrolyte Imbalances (Phosphorus)

Phosphorus, or phosphate, (PO_4) is necessary for neuromuscular and red blood cell function, and the maintenance of acid-base balance, and it provides structure for teeth and bones. About 85% is in the bones, 14% in soft tissue, and less than 1% in ECF. Children have higher levels of phosphorus because of high rate of skeletal growth.

Normal values: 2.5 to 4.5 mg/dL, Hypophosphatemia: less than 2.5 mg/dL, Hyperphosphatemia: more than 4.5 mg/dL.

Hypophosphatemia occurs with severe protein-calorie malnutrition, excess antacids with magnesium or calcium, or albumin, hyperventilation, severe burns, and diabetic ketoacidosis. *Symptoms* include:

irritability, tremors, seizures to coma, hemolytic anemia, decreased myocardial function, respiratory failure. *Treatment:* Identify and treat underlying cause and replace phosphorus.

Hyperphosphatemia occurs with renal failure, hypoparathyroidism, excessive intake, and neoplastic disease, diabetic ketoacidosis, muscle necrosis, and chemotherapy. *Symptoms* include: Tachycardia, muscle cramping, hyperreflexia, and tetany, nausea and diarrhea. *Treatment:* Identify and treat underlying cause, correct hypocalcemia, and provide antacids and dialysis.

Electrolyte Imbalances (Magnesium)

Magnesium (Mg) is the second most common intracellular electrolyte (after potassium) and activates many intracellular enzyme systems. Mg is important for carbohydrate and protein metabolism, neuromuscular function, and cardiovascular function, producing vasodilation and directly affecting the peripheral arterial system:

- Normal values: 1.4 mEq/L.
- Hypomagnesemia: less than 1.4 mEq/L.
- Hypermagnesemia: more than 1.4 mEq/L.

Hypomagnesemia occurs with chronic diarrhea, chronic renal disease, chronic pancreatitis, excess diuretic or laxative use, hyperthyroidism, hypoparathyroidism, severe burns, and diaphoresis. *Symptoms* include:

- neuromuscular excitability/ tetany
- confusion, headaches and dizziness, seizure and coma
- tachycardia with ventricular arrhythmias
- respiratory depression.

Treatment: Identify and treat underlying cause, provide magnesium replacement. *Hypermagnesemia* occurs with renal failure or inadequate renal function, diabetic ketoacidosis, hypothyroidism, and Addison's disease. *Symptoms* include muscle weakness, seizures, dysphagia with decreased gag reflex, and tachycardia with hypotension. *Treatment:* Identify and treat underlying cause, IV hydration with calcium, and dialysis.

Metabolic and Respiratory Acidosis

Comparison of Metabolic and Respiratory Acidosis

Pathophysiology: *Metabolic* -- Increased in fixed acid and inability to excrete acid or loss of base, with compensatory increase of CO_2 excretion by lungs. *Respiratory* -- Hypoventilation and CO_2 retention, with renal compensatory retention of bicarbonate (HCO_3) and increased excretion of hydrogen.

Laboratory: *Metabolic* -- ↓Serum pH and PCO_2 normal if compensated, and↓ if uncompensated. ↓HCO_3. Urine pH < 6 if compensated. *Respiratory* -- ↓Serum pH and ↓PCO_2. HCO_3 normal if compensated and ↓ if uncompensated. Urine pH < 6 if compensated.

Causes: *Metabolic* -- Diabetic ketoacidosis, lactic acidosis, diarrhea, starvation, renal failure, shock, renal tubular acidosis, starvation

Respiratory: COPD, overdose of sedative or barbiturate, obesity, severe pneumonia/atelectasis, muscle weakness (Guillain-Barré), mechanical hypoventilation.

Symptoms: *Metabolic* -- Neuro/muscular: drowsiness, confusion headache, and coma. Cardiac: ↓BP, arrhythmias, flushed skin.

GI: nausea, vomiting, abdominal pain, diarrhea.

Respiratory: Deep inspired tachypnea. *Respiratory* -- Neuro/muscular: drowsiness, dizziness, headache, coma, disorientation, seizures. Cardiac: Flushed skin, ventricular fibrillation, ↓BP, GI: absent. Respiratory: Hypoventilation with hypoxia.

General Issues and Multisystem Problems

Skin Disorders

Burns

Burn injuries may be chemical, electrical, or thermal, and are assessed by the area, percentage of the body burned, and depth:

- *First-degree burns* are superficial and affect the epidermis.
- *Second-degree burns* extend through the dermis (partial thickness).
- *Third-degree burns* affect underlying tissue, including vasculature, muscles, and nerves (full thickness).

Burns are classified according to the American Burn Association's criteria:

- *Minor*
  - less than 10% of body surface area (BSA)
  - 2% BSA with third degree without serious risk to face, hands, feet, or perineum
- *Moderate*
  - 10% to 20% combined second- and third-degree burns, younger than 10 years of age group
  - 10% or less full thickness without serious risk to face, hands, feet, or perineum
- *Major*
  - 20% BSA; at least 10% third-degree burns
  - all burns to face, hands, feet, or perineum that will result in functional/cosmetic defect
  - burns with inhalation or other major trauma

Burn injuries begin with the skin but can affect all organs and body systems, especially with a major burn:

- *Cardiovascular:* Cardiac output may fall by 50% as capillary permeability increases with vasodilation and fluid leaks from the tissues.

- *Urinary:* Decreased blood flow causes kidneys to increase antidiuretic hormone (ADH), which increases oliguria. BUN and creatinine levels increase. Cell destruction may block tubules, and hematuria may result from hemolysis.
- *Pulmonary:* Injury may result from smoke inhalation or (rarely) aspiration of hot liquid. Pulmonary injury is a leading cause of death from burns and is classified according to degree of damage:
  - *First*: Singed eyebrows and nasal hairs with possible soot in airways and slight edema.
  - *Second*: (At 24 hours) Stridor, dyspnea, and tachypnea with edema and erythema of upper airway, including area of vocal chords and epiglottis.
  - *Third*: (At 72 hours) worsening symptoms if not intubated and if intubated, bronchorrhea and tachypnea with edematous, secreting tissue.

Systemic complications of burn injuries include:

- *Neurological:* Encephalopathy may develop from lack of oxygen, decreased blood volume, and sepsis. Hallucinations, alterations in consciousness, seizures, and coma usually result for recovery.
- *GI:* Ileus and ulcerations of mucosa often result from poor circulation. Ileus usually clears within 48 to 72 hours, but if it returns it is often indicative of sepsis.
- *Endocrine/Metabolic:* The sympathetic nervous system stimulates the adrenals to release epinephrine and norepinephrine to increase cardiac output and cortisol for wound healing. The metabolic rate increases markedly. Electrolyte loss occurs with fluid loss from exposed tissue, especially phosphorus, calcium, and sodium, with an increase in potassium levels. Electrolyte imbalance can be life-threatening if burns cover more than 20% of BSA. Glycogen depletion occurs within 12 to 24 hours and protein breakdown, and muscle wasting occurs without sufficient intake of protein.

Management of burn injuries must include both wound care and systemic care to avoid complications that can be life-threatening. Treatment includes:

- Establishment of airway and treatment for inhalation injury as indicated:
- IV fluids and electrolytes, based on weight and extent of burn. Parkland formula: 4 mL/kg/wt x BSA per 24 hours.
- Enteral feedings, usually with small lumen feeding tube into the duodenum.
- NG tube for gastric decompression to prevent aspiration.
- Indwelling catheter to monitor urinary output. Urinary output should be 0.5 to 2 mL/kg/h.
- Analgesia for reduction of pain and anxiety.
- Topical and systemic antibiotics.
- Wound care with removal of eschar and dressings as indicated.

Pressure Ulcers

When assessing an ulcer, it is necessary to determine if it is a non-pressure or pressure ulcer because the treatment protocol may vary depending upon whether the ulcer is caused by pressure, venous or arterial insufficiency, or neuropathic disorders. The clinical basis for this determination should be clearly outlined.

- The ulcer should be classified according to the stage and the characteristics, including size (length, width, and depth).
- Pain associated with the ulcer should be described.
- Photographs should be taken if a protocol is in place.
- Ulcers should be monitored daily and any changes carefully documented.
- The ulcer should be evaluated for signs of infection.

It is important to differentiate between colonization, which is very common, and infection, which usually presents with symptoms such as peri-wound erythema and induration and increased pain, as well as delayed healing of wound. Wound culture and blood tests should be done if there are indications of infection. *Treatment* should be determined according to characteristics of the wound.

The *National Pressure Injury Advisory Panel* developed a staging system to ensure that definitions for pressure ulcers were standardized.

- Stage I: Nonblanchable erythema – Intact, reddened area that does not blanch (Difficult to assess in darker skin). Area remains intact but the physical appearance is altered.
- Stage II: Partial thickness – Destruction of the epidermis and/or dermis. This type of injury may be an intact blister, ruptured blister, or an open ulcer if it has a pinkish or a reddish wound bed.
- Stage III: Full thickness skin loss – Epidermis and dermis have experienced loss and the injury now extends through to the subcutaneous fat tissue. Tunneling could be present. Muscle, tendons, and bones have not been injured.
- Stage IV: Full thickness tissue loss – Damage has progressed to bone, muscle, or tendons. There is often tunneling present, osteomyelitis is common, and the depth of the ulcer will vary by location.
- Unstageable/Unclassified – Injury is present and involves full thickness, but cannot be staged until slough is removed.
- Suspected Deep Tissue Injury – Discolored skin that is still intact but has been damaged. Suspect it is deeper than stage I, but the epidermis is still intact

Contact Dermatitis/Rash

Contact dermatitis is a localized response to contact with an allergen, resulting in a rash that may blister and itch. Common allergens include poison oak, poison ivy, latex, benzocaine, nickel, and preservatives, but there is a wide range of preparations and products to which people may react.

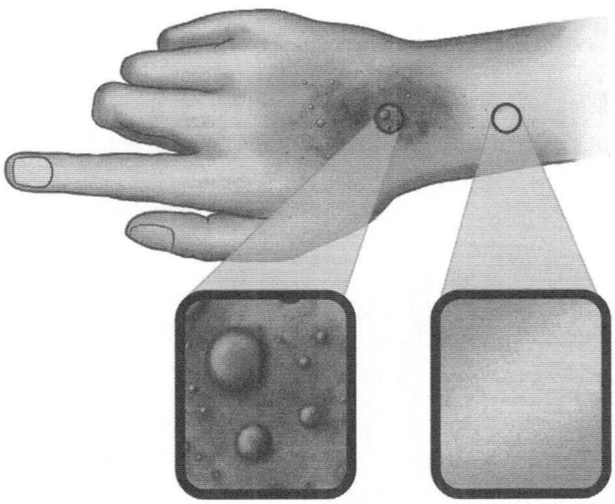

Treatment includes:

- Identifying the causative agent by evaluating the area of the body affected, careful history, or skin patch testing to determine allergic responses.
- Corticosteroids to control inflammation and itching.
- Soothing oatmeal baths.
- Caladryl lotion to relieve itching.
- Antihistamines to reduce allergic response.
- Lesions should be gently cleansed and observed for signs of secondary infection.

- Antibiotics are used only for secondary infections as indicated.
- Rash is usually left open to dry.
- Avoidance of allergen will prevent recurrence.

Toxic Ingestions and Inhalations

Toxic Ingestions/Overdoses

Treatment for toxic ingestions is related to the type of toxin and whether or not it is identified. *Treatment* includes:

- *Administering antidote* if substance is known and an antidote exists. Antidotes for common toxins include:
  - Opiates: naloxone
  - Toxic alcohols: ethanol infusion and/or dialysis
  - Acetaminophen: N-acetylcysteine
  - Calcium channel blockers, beta-blockers: calcium chloride, glucagon.
- *GI decontamination* at one time was standard procedures (ipecac and gastric lavage followed by activated charcoal); it is no longer advised for routine use although selective gastric lavage may be appropriate if done within 1 hour of ingestion.
- *Activated charcoal* (1 g/kg/wt) orally or per NG tube binds to many toxins if given within 1 hour of ingestion. It may also be used in multiple doses (every 4 to 6 hours) to enhance elimination
- *Forced diuresis* with alkalinization of urine (greater than 7.5) may prevent absorption of drugs that are weak bases or acids.

Ethanol Overdose

Ethanol is the form of alcohol found in alcoholic beverages, flavorings, and some medications. It is a multisystem toxin and CNS depressant. Teenagers and younger adults and those older than 60 years of age frequently use ethanol as the drug of choice, but binge drinking can lead to serious morbidity or death. Ethanol has direct effects of the CNS, myocardium, thyroid, and hepatic tissue. Ethanol is absorbed through the mucosa of the mouth, stomach, and intestines, with concentrations peaking about 30 to 60 minutes after ingestion. About 90% of ethanol is metabolized in the liver and the rest excreted through the pulmonary and renal systems. Chronic abuse of ethanol (alcoholism) is also associated with *alcohol withdrawal syndrome (delirium tremens)* with abrupt cessation of alcohol intake, resulting in hallucinations, tachycardia, diaphoresis, and sometimes psychotic behavior. It may be precipitated by trauma or infection and has a high mortality rate, 5% to 15% with treatment and 35% without treatment.

Ethanol overdose affects the CNS as well as other organs in the body. If people are easily aroused, they can usually safely sleep off the effects of ingesting too much alcohol, but if the person is semi-conscious or unconscious, emergency medical treatment should be initiated. Typical *symptoms* include:

- altered mental status with slurred speech and stupor
- nausea and vomiting
- hypotension
- bradycardia with arrhythmias
- respiratory depression and hypoxia
- cold, clammy skin or flushed skin (from vasodilation)
- acute pancreatitis with abdominal pain
- lack of consciousness
- circulatory collapse leading to death.

Treatment includes:

- careful monitoring of arterial blood gases and oxygen saturation
- ensure patent airway with intubation and ventilation if necessary
- IV fluids
- dextrose to correct hypoglycemia if indicated
- maintain body temperature (warming blanket)
- dialysis may be necessary in severe cases.

Inhalation Injuries

Inhalation injuries most often result from exposure to smoke in closed spaces, and often associated with conditions that affect mentation, such as intoxication or head injury. People also often suffer thermal burn injuries. Thermal injuries occur to the upper airway, but inhalation causes injury below the vocal cords. Toxic inhalants can include tissue asphyxiants, pulmonary irritants, and systemic toxins. Patients may suffer from carbon monoxide and hydrogen cyanide poisoning.

Symptoms of inhalation injuries include:

- dyspnea with bronchospasm
- coma from brain hypoxia (carbon monoxide poisoning)
- rapid upper airway edema and delayed (24 hours or less) lower airway edema.

Diagnosis includes clinical examination, ABG and carboxyhemoglobin levels, and chest radiograph,

Treatment includes:

- humidified oxygen, 100%.
- hyperbaric oxygen therapy (carbon monoxide poisoning)
- endotracheal intubation if indicated by severity of burns or respiratory status
- antitoxin therapy according to inhalant.

Acetaminophen Toxicity

Acetaminophen toxicity from accidental or intentional overdose has high rates of morbidity and mortality unless promptly treated. Toxicity occurs with dosage more than 140 mg/kg in one dose or more than 7.5g in 24 hours. *Symptoms* occur in stages:

1. Initial: minor GI upset.
2. Days 2 to 3: hepatotoxicity with right upper quadrant pain and increased AST, ALT, and bilirubin.
3. Days 3 to 4: hepatic failure with metabolic acidosis, coagulopathy, renal failure, encephalopathy, nausea, vomiting, and possible death.
4. Days 5 to 12: recovery period for survivors.

Diagnosis is by history and acetaminophen level, which should be completed within 8 hours of ingestion if possible. Toxicity is plotted on the Rumack-Matthew nomogram with serum levels above 150 requiring antidote. *Treatment* includes:

- GI decontamination with activated charcoal (orally or NG) in patients presenting in less than 24 hours.
- Antidote: 72-hour N-acetylcysteine (NAC) protocol includes 140 mg/kg initially and 70 mg/kg every 4 hours for 17 more doses (orally or IV).
- Supportive therapy.
- The antidote is most effective in 8 hours or less of ingestion but decreases hepatotoxicity even after 24 hours.

Caustic Ingestions

Caustic ingestions of acids (pH less than 7) such as sulfuric, acetic, hydrochloric, and hydrofluoric found in many cleaning agents and alkalis (pH greater than 7) such as sodium hydroxide, potassium hydroxide, sodium tripolyphosphate (in detergents) and sodium hypochlorite (bleach) can result in severe injury and death. Acids cause coagulation necrosis in the esophagus and stomach and may result in metabolic acidosis, hemolysis, and renal failure if systemically absorbed. Alkali injuries cause liquefaction necrosis, resulting in deeper ulcerations, often of the esophagus, but may involve perforation and abdominal necrosis with multiorgan damage. *Symptoms* vary but include pain, dyspnea, oral burns, dysphonia, and vomiting. *Diagnosis:* detailed history, airway examination (oral intubation if possible), ABG, electrolytes, CBC, hepatic and coagulation tests, and radiograph, CT for perforations. *Treatment* includes:

- supportive and symptomatic therapy
- NO ipecac, charcoal, neutralization, or dilution
- NG tube for acids only to aspirate residual
- endoscopy in first few hours to evaluate injury/perforations
- sodium bicarbonate for pH less than 7.10
- prednisolone (alkali injuries).

Amphetamine and Cocaine Toxicity

Amphetamine toxicity may be caused by IV injection, inhalation, or insufflation of various substances, which include methamphetamine (MDA), methylphenidate (Ritalin), methylenedioxymethamphetamine (MDMA or "ecstasy"), and ephedrine and phenylpropanolamine. Cocaine may be ingested orally, IV, or by insufflation, while crack cocaine may be smoked. Amphetamines and cocaine are CNS stimulants that can cause multisystem abnormalities. Symptoms may include chest pain, dysrhythmias, myocardial ischemia, MI, seizures, intracranial infarctions, hypertension, dystonia, repetitive movements, unilateral blindness, lethargy, rhabdomyolysis with acute kidney failure, perforated nasal septum (cocaine), and paranoid psychosis (amphetamines). Crack cocaine may cause pulmonary hemorrhage, asthma, pulmonary edema, barotrauma, and pneumothorax. Swallowing packs of cocaine can cause intestinal ischemia, colitis, necrosis, and perforation. Diagnosis includes clinical findings, CBC, chemistry panel, toxicology screening, ECG, radiograph.

Treatment includes: gastric emptying (1 hour or less), charcoal administration, IV access, supplemental oxygen sedation for seizures: Lorazepam 2 mg, diazepam 5 mg IV titrated in repeated doses, agitation: haloperidol, hypertension: nitroprusside, phentolamine 2.5 to 5 mg IV, cocaine quinidine-like effects: sodium bicarbonate.

Acute Pancreatitis

Acute pancreatitis is related to chronic alcoholism or cholelithiasis in 90% of patients. Pancreatitis may be triggered by a variety of drugs. Pain is usually acute and may be mid-epigastric, left upper abdominal, or more generalized. Nausea and vomiting, as well as Abdominal distension may be present. Complications may include shock, acute respiratory distress syndrome, and multiorgan failure. *Diagnostic* tests include:

- serum lipase greater than 2 times normal value
- serum amylase (less accurate than lipase)
- CT with contrast to determine if there is pancreatic necrosis
- ultrasound to check bile duct for obstruction
- magnetic resonance (MR) cholangiopancreatography may be used in place of CT and ultrasound where available.

Treatment is usually supportive with oral intake restricted to clear liquids. Rehydration with IV fluids may be needed. Biliary obstruction needs to be removed with cholecystectomy. Antibiotics are given if necrosis is related to infection. Analgesia may be indicated.

Pharmacology

Digitalis

Digitalis drugs, most commonly administered in the form of digoxin, are derived from the foxglove plant and are used to increase myocardial contractility, left ventricular output, and slow conduction through the atrioventricular (AV) node, decreasing rapid heart rates and promoting diuresis. Digoxin does not affect mortality, but increases tolerance to activity and reduces hospitalizations for heart failure. Therapeutic levels (0.5 to 2 ng/mL) should be maintained to avoid digitalis toxicity, which can occur even if digoxin levels are within the therapeutic range, so observation of symptoms is critical. Potassium imbalance may cause toxicity.

Evidence of toxicity includes:

- Early signs: increasing fatigue, lethargy, depression, and nausea and vomiting.
- Sudden change in heart rhythm, such as regular or irregular rhythm.
- Sinoatrial (SA) or AV block, new ventricular dysrhythmias, and tachycardia (atrial, junctional, and/or ventricular).

Treatment of digitalis toxicity involves discontinuing medication and monitoring serum levels and symptoms. Digoxin immune FAB may be used to bind to digoxin and inactivate it if necessary.

Heart Failure and Hypertension

There are a number of different types of medications used for the treatment of heart failure and hypertension:

- *Ace inhibitors,* such as captopril, enalapril, and lisinopril, decrease afterload and preload and reverse ventricular remodeling but may cause hypotension initially and are contraindicated with renal insufficiency.
- Angiotensin receptor blockers
- *Beta-blockers,* such as metoprolol, carvedilol, and esmolol, slow the heart rate, reduce hypertension, prevent dysrhythmias, and reverse ventricular remodeling, but should not be used during decompensation and should be monitored carefully for those with airway disease, uncontrolled diabetes, slow irregular pulse, or heart block.
- *Aldosterone antagonists,* such as spironolactone (Aldactone), reduce preload, myocardial hypertrophy, and edema. These drugs may increase blood levels of potassium because this is a potassium-sparing diuretic. Therefore, while water and sodium are excreted, potassium is retained.

Vasodilators (Smooth Muscle Relaxants)

Vasodilators may be used for arterial dilation or venous dilation in order to improve cardiac function. These drugs may be used to treat pulmonary hypertension or generalized systemic hypertension. They may be used for those who cannot tolerate ACE inhibitors or angiotensin receptor blockers. Vasodilators may dilate arteries, veins, or both.

- Arterial dilation reduces afterload, improving cardiac output.
- Venous dilation reduces preload, reducing filling pressures.

There are numerous types of vasodilators:

- *Smooth muscle relaxants* decrease peripheral vascular resistance but may cause hypotension and headaches:
  - Sodium nitroprusside (Nipride®) dilates both arteries and veins. It is rapid in action and used for reduction of hypertension and afterload reduction for heart failure.
  - Nitroglycerin (Tridil®) primarily dilates veins and is used IV to reduce preload for acute heart failure, unstable angina, and acute MI. Nitroglycerin may also be prophylactically after PCIs to prevent vasospasm.

- *Hydralazine (Apresoline®)* dilates arteries and is given intermittently to reduce hypertension.
- *Calciumchannel blockers* are primarily arterial vasodilators that may affect the peripheral and/or coronary arteries. Side effects include lethargy, flushing, abdominal and peripheral edema, and indigestion:
  - Dihydropyridine calcium channel blockers, such as nifedipine and nicardipine (Cardene®), are primarily arterial vasodilators affecting both coronary and peripheral arteries. They are used to treat acute hypertension.
  - Benzothiazine derivatives, such as diltiazem (Cardizem®) and phenylalkylamine such as verapamil (Calan®, Isoptin®), dilate primarily coronary arteries and are used for angina and supraventricular tachycardias.
- *Angiotensin-converting enzyme (ACE) inhibitors* limit production of the peripheral vasoconstricting angiotensin, resulting in vasodilation, which can cause a precipitous fall in blood pressure, so use must be carefully monitored. They are often the first line of drugs to be used for acute hypertension and heart failure and are used to prevent nephropathy in patients with diabetes: Captopril (Capoten®) and enalapril (Vasotec®) decrease afterload and preload for heart failure.
- *B-type natriuretic (BNP) peptide,* such as nesiritide (Natrecor®), is a new type of vasodilator, which is a recombinant form of a peptide of the human brain. It decreases filling pressure and vascular resistance, and increases urinary output, but may cause hypotension, headache, bradycardia, and nausea.
- *Alpha-adrenergic blockers* block alpha receptors in arteries and veins, causing vasodilation. However, it may also cause orthostatic hypotension and edema from fluid retention:
  - Labetalol (Normodyne®) is a combination peripheral alpha-blocker and cardiac beta-blocker and is used to treat acute hypertension, acute stroke, and acute aortic dissection.
  - Phentolamine (Regitine®) is a peripheral arterial dilator that reduces afterload and is used for pheochromocytoma.
- *Selective specific dopamine DA-1 receptor agonists,* such as fenoldopam (Corlopam®), are peripheral dilators affecting renal and mesenteric arteries and can be used for patients with renal dysfunction or those at risk of renal insufficiency.

ANTIDYSRHYTHMICS

Antidysrhythmics include a number of drugs that act on the conduction system, the ventricles, and/or the atria to control dysrhythmias. There are 4 classes of drugs that are used as well as some that are unclassified:

- Class I: 3 subtypes of sodium channel blockers (quinidine, lidocaine, procainamide)
- Class II: beta-receptor blockers (esmolol, propranolol)
- Class III: slows repolarization (amiodarone, ibutilide)
- Class IV: calcium channel blockers (diltiazem, verapamil)
- Unclassified (adenosine).

DYSRHYTHMIAS

Supraventricular tachycardia:

- Adenosine affects the conduction system and may cause transient flushing, decreased BP, and shortness of breath.
- Diltiazem (Cardizem®, Tiazac®) affects the conduction system and may cause bradycardia, AV block, and decreased BP.
- Esmolol (Brevibloc®) affects the conduction system and may cause decreased BP, bradycardia, and heart failure.
- Propranolol (Inderal®) affects the conduction system and may cause bradycardia, heart block, and heart failure.

- Procainamide affects the atria and ventricles and may cause decreased BP and ECG abnormalities (widening of QRS and QT).
- Paroxysmal supraventricular tachycardia: Adenosine; Digoxin (Lanoxin®) affects the conduction system and may cause bradycardia, heart block, nausea and vomiting, and CNS depression; Verapamil (Calan®, Verelan®) affects the conduction system and may cause decreased BP, bradycardia, and heart failure.
- Atrial fibrillation: Digoxin (Lanoxin®), Diltiazem (Cardizem®, Tiazac®); Ibutilide (Corvert®) affects the conduction system and rarely has side effects; Amiodarone (Cordarone®) affects the atria and ventricles and may cause decreased BP and adverse hepatic effects.
- Atrial flutter: Digoxin (Lanoxin®), Diltiazem (Cardizem®, Tiazac®), Ibutilide (Corvert®), Verapamil (Calan®, Verelan®), Amiodarone (Cordarone®), Procainamide.
- Sinus tachycardia: Esmolol (Brevibloc®).
- Premature ventricular contractions: Lidocaine affects the ventricles and may cause CNS toxicity with nausea and vomiting; Procainamide.
- Ventricular tachycardia: Lidocaine, Amiodarone (Cardizem®, Tiazac®), Procainamide.
- Ventricular fibrillation: Lidocaine.

Loop Diuretics

Diuretics increase renal perfusion and filtration, thereby reducing preload and decreasing peripheral and pulmonary edema, hypertension, CHF, diabetes insipidus, and osteoporosis. There are different types of diuretics: loop, thiazide, and potassium sparing.

Loop diuretics inhibit the reabsorption of sodium and chloride (primarily) in the ascending loop of Henle. They also cause increased secretion of other electrolytes, such as calcium, magnesium, and potassium, and this can result in imbalances that cause dysrhythmias. Other side effects include frequent urination, postural hypotension, and increased blood sugar and uric acid levels. They are short-acting, which means they are less effective than other diuretics for control of hypertension:

- *Bumetanide* (Bumex®) is given intravenously after surgery to reduce preload or orally to treat heart failure.
- *Ethacrynic acid* (Edecrin®) is given intravenously after surgery to reduce preload.
- *Furosemide* (Lasix®) is used for the control of (CHF) congestive heart failure as well as renal insufficiency. It is used after surgery to decrease preload and to reduce the inflammatory response caused by cardiopulmonary bypass (postperfusion syndrome).

Thiazide Diuretics

Thiazide diuretics inhibit the reabsorption of sodium and chloride primarily in the early distal tubules, forcing more sodium and water to be excreted. Thiazide diuretics increase secretion of potassium and bicarbonate, so they are often given with supplementary potassium or in combination with potassium-sparing diuretics. Thiazide diuretics are the first line of drugs for treatment of hypertension. They have a long duration of action (12 to 72 hours, depending on the drug) so they are able to maintain control of hypertension better than short-acting drugs. They may be given daily or 3 to 5 days per week. There are numerous thiazide diuretics, including:

- chlorothiazide(Diuril®)
- bendroflumethiazide(Naturetin®)
- chlorthalidone(Hygroton)
- Trichlormethiazide.(Naqua®)

Side effects include dizziness, light-headedness, postural hypotension, headache, blurred vision, and itching, especially during initial treatment. Thiazide diuretics cause sensitivity to sun exposure, so people should be counseled to use sunscreen

Potassium-Sparing Diuretics

Potassium-sparing diuretics inhibit the reabsorption of sodium in the late distal tubule and collecting duct. They are weaker than thiazide or loop diuretics, but do not cause a reduction in potassium level; however, if used alone, they may cause an increase in potassium, which can cause weakness, irregular pulse, and cardiac arrest. Because potassium-sparing diuretics are less effective alone, they are often given in a combined form with a thiazide diuretic (usually chlorothiazide), which mitigates the potassium imbalance.

Typical side effects include dehydration, blurred vision, nausea insomnia, and nasal congestion, especially in the first few days of treatment:

- *Spironolactone* (Aldactone®) is a synthetic steroid diuretic that increases the secretion of both water and sodium and is used to treat congestive heart failure. It may be given orally or IV.
- *Eplerenone* is similar to spironolactone but has fewer side effects so it may be used with patients who cannot tolerate the other drug.

Asthma

Numerous pharmacological agents are used for control of asthma, some long acting to prevent attacks and others that are short-acting to provide relief for acute episodes:

- *Beta-adrenergic agonists* include both long-acting and short-acting preparations used for relaxation of smooth muscles and bronchodilation, reducing edema and aiding clearance of mucus. Medications include salmeterol (Serevent®), sustained-release albuterol (Volmax ER®) and short-acting albuterol (Proventil®) and levalbuterol (Xopenex®).
- *Anticholinergics* aid in preventing bronchial constriction and potentiate the bronchodilating action of beta-adrenergic agonists. The most-commonly used medication is ipratropium bromide (Atrovent®).
- *Corticosteroids* provide anti-inflammatory action by inhibiting immune responses, decreasing edema, mucus, and hyperresponsiveness. Because of numerous side effects, glucocorticosteroid are usually administered orally or parentally for 5 days (prednisone, prednisolone, methylprednisolone) and then the patient is switched to inhaled steroids. If a patient receives glucocorticoids for more than 5 days, then dosages are tapered. Inhaled corticosteroids include beclomethasone (Vanceril®), budesonide (Pulmicort®) and fluticasone propionate (Flovent®).
- *Methylxanthines* are generally contraindicated for children unless the child is critically ill, in which case they appear to have a role in improving pulmonary function and decreasing the need for mechanical ventilation. Medications include aminophylline and theophylline.
- *Magnesium sulfate* is used to relax smooth muscles and decrease inflammation. If administered intravenously, it must be given slowly to prevent hypotension and bradycardia. Inhaled, it potentiates the action of albuterol.
- *Heliox* (helium-oxygen) is administered to decrease airway resistance with airway obstruction, thereby decreasing respiratory effort. Heliox improves oxygenation of patients on mechanical ventilation.
- *Leukotriene inhibitors* are used to inhibit inflammation and bronchospasm for long-term management. Medications include montelukast (Singulair®).

Pulmonary Pharmacology

There are a wide range of agents used for **pulmonary pharmacology**, depending upon the type and degree of pulmonary disease. Agents include:

- **Opioid analgesics:** Used to provide both pain relief and sedation for those on mechanical ventilation to reduce sympathetic response. Medications may include fentanyl (Sublimaze®) or morphine sulfate (MS Contin®).

- **Neuromuscular blockers:** Used for induced paralysis of those who have not responded adequately to sedation, especially for intubation and mechanical ventilation. Medications may include pancuronium (Pavulon®) and vecuronium (Norcuron®). However, there is controversy about the use as induced paralysis has been linked to increased mortality rates, sensory hearing loss (pancuronium), atelectasis, and ventilation-perfusion mismatch.
- **Human B-type natriuretic peptides:** Used to reduce pulmonary capillary wedge pressure. Medications include nesiritide (Natrecor®).
- ***Vasopressors/Inotropes:*** Used to increase cardiac output. Dopamine increases renal output and blood pressure. Dobutamine increases cardiac contractibility and blood pressure.
- ***Surfactants****:* Reduces surface tension to prevent collapse of alveoli. Beractant is derived from bovine lung tissue and calfactant from calf lung tissue. They are administered as inhalants.
- ***Alkalinizers***: Used to treat metabolic acidosis and decrease pulmonary vascular resistance by achieving an alkaline pH. Medications include sodium bicarbonate and tromethamine.
- ***Pulmonary vasodilator (inhaled nitrous oxide):*** Used to relax the vascular muscles and produce pulmonary vasodilation. Some studies show it reduces need for extracorporeal membrane oxygenation (ECMO), although this is not supported by other studies.
- ***Methylxanthines***: Used to stimulate muscle contractions of chest and stimulate respirations. Medications include aminophylline, caffeine citrate, and doxapram.
- ***Diuretis****:* Used to reduce pulmonary edema. Medications include loop diuretics such as furosemide (Lasix®) and metolazone (Mykrox®).
- ***Nitrates****:* Used for vasodilation to reduce preload and afterload to reduce myocardial need for oxygen. Medications include nitroglycerin (Nitro-Bid®) and nitroprusside sodium (Nitropress®).
- ***Antibiotics****:* Used for treatment of respiratory infections, including pneumonia. Medications are used according to the pathogenic agent and may include macrolides, such as azithromycin (Zithromax®) and erythromycin (E-Mycin®).
- ***Antimycobacterials****:* Used for treatment of tuberculosis (TB) and other mycobacterial diseases. Medications include isoniazid (Laniazid®, Nydrazid®), ethambutol (Myambutol®), rifampin (Rifadin®), streptomycin sulfate, and pyrazinamide.
- ***Antivirals****:* Used to inhibit replication of virus early in a viral infection. Effectiveness decreases as time passes because replication process has already begun. Medications include ribavirin (Virazole®) and zanamivir (Relenza®).

Advocacy/Moral Agency

Assessing Issues

While the terms *ethics* and *morals* are sometimes used interchangeably, ethics is a study of morals and encompasses concepts of right and wrong. When making ethical assessments, one must consider not only what people should do but what they actually do, as these two things are sometimes at odds. Ethical issues can be difficult to assess because of personal bias, and that is one of the reasons that sharing concerns with other internal sources and reaching consensus is so valuable. Issues of concern might include options for care, refusal of care, rights to privacy, adequate relief of suffering, and the right to self-determination. Internal sources might include the ethics committee, whose charge is to make decisions regarding ethical issues. Risk management can provide guidance related to personal and institutional liability. External agencies might include government agencies, such as the public health department.

Organizational Ethics

Organizational ethics is the value system at work within an organization. While almost all health care organizations have a Code of Ethics, an ethical organization embodies that code within all processes, including:

- Relationships with customers and the public, utilizing a code of right conduct.
- Recognition of the patient's/customer's right to quality care, and respect for personal religious beliefs, culture, and psychosocial values.
- Openness in disclosure of information and accountability.
- Adherence to regulations and best practices.
- Recognition of the need to empower staff and patients/customers.
- Leadership without intimidation or fear tactics.
- Following standard open guidelines for organ donation and procurement and for research projects.
- Maintenance of a bioethics committee to provide guidance related to ethical issues in health care.

Beneficence and Nonmaleficence

Beneficence is an ethical principle that involves performing actions that are for the purpose of benefiting another person. In the care of a patient, any procedure or treatment should be done with the ultimate goal of benefiting the patient, and any actions that are not beneficial should be reconsidered. As a child ages and/or condition changes, procedures need to be continually reevaluated to determine if they are still of benefit.

Nonmaleficence is an ethical principle that means health care workers should provide care in a manner that does not cause direct intentional harm to the patient:

- The actual act must be good or morally neutral.
- The intent must be only for a good effect.
- A bad effect cannot serve as the means to get to a good effect.
- A good effect must have more benefit than a bad effect has harm.

Autonomy and Justice

Autonomy is the ethical principle that the individual has the right to make decisions about his or her own care. In the case of children, the child cannot make autonomous decisions, so the parents serve as the legal decision maker. The nurse must keep the parents fully informed so that they can exercise their autonomy in informed decision making. *Justice* is the ethical principle that relates to the distribution of the limited resources of health care benefits to the members of society. These resources must be distributed fairly. This issue may arise if there is only one bed left and two sick children. Justice comes into play in deciding which child should stay and which should be transported or otherwise cared for. The decision should be made according to what is best or most just for the patients and not colored by personal bias.

BIOETHICS

Bioethics is a branch of ethics that involves making sure that the medical treatment given is the most morally correct choice given the different options that might be available and the differences inherent in the varied levels of treatment. In the acute/critical care unit, if the patients, parents, and the staff are in agreement when it comes to values and decision making, then no ethical dilemma exists; however, when there is a difference in value beliefs between the patients/parents and the staff, there is a bioethical dilemma that must be resolved. Sometimes, discussion and explanation can resolve differences, but at times the institution's ethics committee must be brought in to resolve the conflict. The primary goal of bioethics is to determine the most morally correct action using the set of circumstances given.

PATIENT/FAMILY RIGHTS

In order for patient/family rights to be incorporated into the plan of care, the care plan needs to be designed as a collaborative effort that encourages participation of patients and family members. There are a number of different programs that can be useful, such as including patients and families on advisory committees. Additionally, assessment tools, such as surveys for patients/families, can be utilized to gain insight in the issues that are important to them. While infants and small children and sometimes elderly patients cannot speak for themselves, "patient" is generally understood to include not only the immediate family but also other groups or communities who have an interest in the care of an individual or individuals. Because many hospital stays are now short-term, programs that include follow-up interviews and assessments are especially valuable in determining if the needs of the patient/family were addressed in the care plan.

INTEGRATING CONCERNS

Integrating the concerns and value systems of the patient/family, nursing staff, other health care team members, administrators and into patient's plan of care requires a determination and understanding of what is important to each participant. Planning for this type of integration is an ongoing effort as it is not practical to call a participant meeting to discuss each care plan, but general concerns and values can be identified for the institution or the unit and these can then be individualized for each patient. Participants may have widely divergent concerns. For example:

- A child may want her parents to be with her at all times.
- A parent may want religious/cultural concerns about medical care to be respected.
- A payor may want appropriate and cost-effective treatments.
- A nurse may want treatments to be clearly outlined and carried out competently.
- A nutritionist may want the child to have adequate nutrition.
- An adequate care plan should allow for all of these concerns to be addressed.

ETHICAL DECISION MAKING

An environment for ethical decision making and patient advocacy does not appear when it is needed; it requires planning and preparation. The expectation for the institution should clearly communicate that nurses are legally and morally responsible for ensuring competent care and respecting the rights of patients. Decisions regarding ethical issues often must be made quickly with little time for contemplation; therefore, ethical issues that may arise should be identified and discussed. Clearly defined procedures and policies for dealing with conflicts, including an active ethics committee, inservice training, and staff meetings, must be established. Patients and families need to be part of the ethical environment, and that means empowering them by providing patient/family information (print form, video, audio) that outlines the patient's rights and procedures for expressing their wishes and dealing with ethical conflicts. Respect for privacy and confidentiality and a nonpunitive atmosphere are essential.

CONFIDENTIALITY

Confidentiality is the obligation that is present in a professional-patient relationship. Nurses are under an obligation to protect the information they possess concerning the patient and family. Care should be taken to safeguard that information and provide the privacy that the family deserves. This is accomplished through the use of required passwords when family calls for information about the patient and through the limitation of who is allowed to visit. There may be times when confidentiality must be broken to save the life of a patient, but those circumstances are rare. The nurse practitioner must make all efforts to safeguard patient records and identification. Computerized record keeping should be done in such a way that the screen is not visible to others, and paper records must be secured.

Minors, especially adolescents, may have areas of concern in relation to their health or activities that they do not want divulged to their parents. Young people may be uncomfortable addressing concerns verbally and may be more forthcoming if given a questionnaire to fill out as a beginning point for discussion. The acute care nurse is often faced with ethical concerns about dealing with confidentiality, but the best course is to deal with the issue directly by informing adolescents that what they say will be held in confidence within certain limitations:

- Mandatory reporting requirements must be upheld, including reports of child abuse, sexual abuse, and communicable diseases.
- Health endangerment, such as through the abuse of drugs or alcohol, eating disorders, or suicidal thoughts, must be reported to the parents, while assuring the child that the acute care nurse will be there to support and help them to discuss these matters with parents.

Informed Consent

Patients or guardians must provide informed consent for all treatment the patient receives. This includes a thorough explanation of all procedures and treatment and associated risks. Patients/guardians should be apprised of all options and allowed input on the type of treatments. Patients/guardians should be apprised of all reasonable risks and any complications that might be life-threatening or increase morbidity. The American Medical Association has established guidelines for informed consent:

- explanation of diagnosis
- Nature of, and reason for, treatment or procedure
- risks and benefits
- alternative options (regardless of cost or insurance coverage)
- risks and benefits of alternative options
- risks and benefits of not having a treatment or procedure.
- Providing informed consent is a requirement of all states.

Children and adolescents younger than 18 years of age (minors), unless legally emancipated, lack the legal right to give consent for medical treatments until they reach the age of majority except in those areas approved by law, such as for birth control, abortion, and HIV testing, and even these vary from one state to another, with some requiring parent notification. However, children must be included in discussions about treatment options in accordance to their age and level of understanding. Because children do not always appreciate cause/effect relationships, the law allows the parents to override decisions of the child and teenager, but forcing the child to have treatment puts the child in a poor emotional state for healing and is cause for ethical concern. Therefore, the nurse practitioner should work with both the parents and the child, explaining the benefits and disadvantages of treatment, to try to bring about agreement or assent on the part of the child. This is especially important for adolescents, who are seeking autonomy. Discussions about when to stop treatment and advance directives should include the child whenever possible.

Ethical and Clinical Conflicts

Ethical and clinical conflicts among patients and their families and health care providers are not uncommon. Issues frequently relate to medications and treatment, religion, concepts of truth telling, lack of respect for patient's autonomy, and limitations of managed care or incompetent care. Additionally, health care providers are in a position to easily manipulate patients/families by providing incomplete information to influence decisions, and this can give rise to ethical conflicts. Facilitation involves questioning and listening, and acknowledging each person's perspective while sharing different viewpoints:

- Open communication is critical to solving conflicts. Asking what steps could be taken to resolve the conflict or how it could be handled differently often leads to compromise because it allows for exchange of ideas and validates legitimate concerns. Sharing cultural perspectives can lead to better understanding.
- Advocacy for the patients/families must remain at the center of conflict resolution.

Child Abuse

About 5 million cases of suspected child abuse are reported in the United States each year. In accordance with the Child Abuse Prevention and Treatment Act Amendments (1996) and the Model Child Protection Act, all states have instituted mandatory reporting of child abuse. The acute care nurse practitioner should be knowledgeable about the statutes in the state of practice, but medical personnel are mandatory reporters and must report the following:

- Child abuse or neglect that places the child in risk of harm (physical or emotional), death, or exploitation.
- Sexual abuse, including rape, molestation, prostitution, incest, or coercion to engage in any type of sexually explicit behavior.

While some statutes mandate reporting of suspicion, others mandate more knowledge; however, there is criminal and civil liability involved if child abuse is not reported and most states provide immunity for reporters, so the best course is to report suspicions to child protective services or the police, according to the state requirements.

Genetic Testing

Genetic testing poses a number of ethical issues because parents can authorize genetic testing without the consent of the minor. The acute care nurse practitioner must serve as an advocate for the child/adolescent in cases in which genetic testing is done to determine if the child is a carrier or has an adult-onset genetic disease for which there is no cure or adequate treatment, such as Huntington disease. In both of these cases, the information derived from testing cannot be used for health promotion or disease prevention, so the parents should be counseled to wait until the child is at least in the teen years and can make an informed decision about whether to have testing. This type of information can be devastating to young people who are not provided adequate support and counseling prior to testing. Some people with adult-onset diseases choose not to be tested, and childhood testing robs them of this choice.

Approaches Aiding Advocacy

There are a number of different approaches that can help develop nurses' advocacy and moral agency:

- *Role modeling* takes place when one nurse serves as a role for others, modeling the behavior and responses that advocate for the patient and show caring practices.
- *Modeling and role modeling* is another concept that is particularly useful in the development of ethical practices. In this case, modeling occurs when the nurse, through observation and interviewing, attempts to gain an understanding of the patient/family's perspective. Then the role modeling uses that understanding to assist the patient/family by intervening to ensure that their needs are met.
- *Coaching* involves providing staff with tools, ways to respond or procedures to follow, to help them to understand how they can become an advocate.
- *Mentoring* is providing professional guidance, someone to whom a staff person can bring questions or concerns.

Empowering patients and families to act as their own advocates requires they have a clear understanding of their rights and responsibilities. These should be given (in print form) and/or presented (audio/video) to patients and families on admission or as soon as possible:

- *Rights* should include competent, nondiscriminatory medical care that respects privacy and allows participation in decisions about care and the right to refuse care. They should have clear, understandable explanations of treatments, options, and conditions, including outcomes. They should be apprised of transfers, changes in care plan, and advance directives. They should have access to medical records' information about charges.
- *Responsibilities* should include providing honest and thorough information about health issues and medical history. They should ask for clarification if they do not understand information that is provided to them, and they should follow the plan of care that is outlined or explain why that is not possible. They should treat staff and other patients with respect.

Terminally Ill Patients

There are a number of ethical concerns that health care providers and families must face when determining the treatments that are necessary and appropriate for a terminally ill patient. It is the nurse's responsibility to provide support and information to help parents/families make informed decisions:

- *Pain medications: Advantages* -- Provide comfort. Ease the dying process. *Disadvantages* -- Increase sedation and decrease cognition and interaction with family. Side effects. May hasten death.
- *Active treatments (e.g., antibiotics, chemotherapy): Advantages* -- Prolong life. Relieve symptoms. Reassure family. *Disadvantages* -- Prolong the dying process. Side effects may be severe (as with chemotherapy).
- *Supplemental nutrition: Advantages* -- Relieve family's anxiety that child is hungry. Prolong life. *Disadvantages* -- May cause nausea, vomiting. May increase tumor growth with cancer. May increase discomfort. May cause nausea, vomiting. May increase tumor growth with cancer. May increase discomfort.
- *IV fluids for hydration: Advantages* -- Relieve family's anxiety that child is thirsty. Keep mouth moist. *Disadvantages* --May result in congestive heart failure and pulmonary edema with increased dyspnea. Increased urinary output and incontinence may cause skin breakdown. Prolong dying process.
- *Resuscitation efforts: Advantages* -- Allow family to deny death is imminent. *Disadvantages* -- Cause unnecessary suffering and prolong dying process.

Problem Solving

The importance of problem solving to anticipate and prevent recurrences of patient/family dissatisfaction or concern.

- Problem solving to anticipate or prevent recurrences of patient/family dissatisfaction involves arriving at a hypothesis, testing, and assessing data to determine if the hypothesis holds true. If a problem has arisen, taking steps to resolve the immediate problem is only the first step if recurrence is to be avoided:
- *The issue*: Talk with the patient or family and staff to determine if the problem is related to a failure of communication or other issues, such as culture or religion.
- *Collect data*: This may mean interviewing additional staff or reviewing documentation, gaining a variety of perspectives.
- *Important concepts*: Determine if there are issues related to values or beliefs.
- *Consider reasons for actions*: Distinguish between motivation and intention on the part of all parties to determine the reason for the problem.
- *Make a decision*: A decision on how to prevent a recurrence of a problem should be based on advocacy and moral agency, reaching the best solution possible for the patient and family.

Patients' Rights

Patients' (families') rights in relation to what they should expect from a health care organization are outlined in both standards of the Joint Commission and National Committee for Quality Assurance. Rights include:

- Respect for patient, including personal dignity and psychosocial, spiritual, and cultural considerations.
- Response to needs related to access and pain control.
- Ability to make decisions about care, including informed consent, advance directives, and end-of-life care.
- Procedure for registering complaints or grievances.
- Protection of confidentiality and privacy.
- Freedom from abuse or neglect.
- Protection during research and information related to ethical issues of research.
- Appraisal of outcomes, including unexpected outcomes.
- Information about organization, services, and practitioners.
- Appeal procedures for decisions regarding benefits and quality of care.
- Organizational code of ethical behavior.
- Procedures for donating and procuring organs/tissue.

Safe Passage

Facilitating safe passage is part of caring practice that ensures patient safety, in a broad sense, from a variety of perspectives:

- Giving appropriate medications and treatment without errors that endanger the child's health is essential.
- Providing information to the patient/family about treatments, changes, conditions, and other aspects related to care helps them to cope with the situations as they arise.
- Preventing infection is central to patient safety and includes staff using proper infection control methods, such as handwashing.
- Knowing the person requires the nurse to take the time and effort to understand the needs and wishes of the patient/family.

Assisting with transitions involves not only helping the patient/family cope with moving from one form of treatment, or one unit to another, but also with transitions in health, such as from illness to health or from illness to death.

Advance Directives

In accordance to federal and state laws, individuals have the right to self-determination in health care, including decisions about end-of-life care through advance directives such as living wills and the right to assign a surrogate person to make decisions through a durable power of attorney. Patients should routinely be questioned about an advance directive as they may present to a health care provider without the document. Patients who have indicated they desire a DNR order should not receive resuscitative treatments for terminal illness or conditions in which meaningful recovery cannot occur. Patients and families of those with terminal illnesses should be questioned as to whether the patients are hospice patients. For those with DNR requests or those withdrawing life support, staff should provide the patient palliative rather than curative measures, such as pain control and/or oxygen, and emotional support to the patient and family. Religious traditions and beliefs about death should be treated with respect.

End-of-Life Palliative Care

The World Health Organization (WHO) defines end-of-life and palliative care as active total care of a patient whose disease is no longer responsive to treatment. Palliative care, especially pain management, is often delayed or inadequate in patients. The dying patient and family must be considered a unit when planning for care, and a multidisciplinary approach that includes physicians, nurses, social workers, and chaplains or spiritual guides can help the family through this difficult period. Family may equate pain medication with euthanasia or assisted suicide. Additionally, the family may feel that the patient's increased sedation robs them of time with the patient or may fear addiction. These concerns must be respected, but providing adequate information and support while allowing the parents/family to express their feelings can often allay many of these fears.

Support Before Death

Families of dying patients often do not receive adequate support from nursing staff, who feel unprepared for dealing with their grief and unsure of how to provide comfort. Families may be in desperate need of this support:

Before death	Stay with the family and sit quietly, allowing them to talk, cry, or interact if they desire.
	Avoid platitudes, "His suffering will be over soon."
	Avoid judgmental reactions to what family members say or do and realize that anger, fear, guilt, and irrational behavior are normal responses to acute grief and stress.
	Show caring by touching the patient and encouraging family to do the same. Note: Touching hands, arms, or shoulders of family members can provide comfort, but follow clues of the family.
	Provide referrals to support groups if available.

Support When Patient Dies

The family requires much support when the patient dies:

Time of death	Reassure family that all measures have been taken to ensure the patient's comfort. Express personal feeling of loss, "She was such a sweet woman, and I'll miss her," and allow family to express feelings and memories. Provide information about what is happening during the dying process, explaining death rales, Cheyne-Stokes respirations, etc.
	Alert family members to imminent death if they are not present. Assist to contact clergy/spiritual advisors.
	Respect feelings and needs of parents, siblings, and other family.
After death	Encourage parents/family members to stay with the patient as long as they wish to say goodbye.
	Use the patient's name when talking to the family.
	Assist family to make arrangements, such as contacting funeral home. If an autopsy is required, discuss with the family and explain when it will take place. If organ donation is to occur, assist the family to make arrangements. Encourage family members to grieve and express emotions. Send card or condolence note.

Stages of Grief

Grief is a normal response to the death or severe illness/abnormality of a patient. How a person deals with grief is very personal, and each will grieve differently. Elisabeth Kübler-Ross identified five stages of grief in

On Death and Dying (1969), which can apply to both patients and family members. A person may not go through each stage but usually goes through two of the five stages:

- Denial: Patients/families may be resistive to information and unable to accept that a person is dying/impaired. They may act stunned, immobile, or detached and may be unable to respond appropriately or remember what is said, often repeatedly asking the same questions.
- Anger: As reality becomes clear, patient/families may react with pronounced anger, directed inward or outward. Women, especially, may blame themselves and self-anger may lead to severe depression and guilt, assuming they are to blame because of some personal action. Outward anger, more common in men, may be expressed as overt hostility.
- Bargaining: This involves if-then thinking (often directed at a deity): "If I go to church every way, then God will prevent this." Patient/family may change doctors, trying to change the outcome.
- Depression: As the patient and family begin to accept the loss, they may become depressed, feeling no one understands, and overwhelmed with sadness. They may be tearful or crying and may withdraw or ask to be left alone.
- Acceptance: This final stage represents a form of resolution and often occurs outside of the medical environment after months. Patients are able to accept death/dying/incapacity. Families are able to resume their normal activities and lose the constant preoccupation with their loved one. They are able to think of the person without severe pain.

Types of Family Grief

Anticipatory grief occurs when a person is diagnosed with a terminal illness. The family begins to mourn over the loss of the person before he or she expires.

Incongruent grief occurs when family members, such as the mother and the father, are "out of synch" in their grieving process, stressing their relationship. It may be due to the differences in how men and women grieve, or it may be because the dynamics between the patient and the family members are different.

Delayed grief occurs when the grieving process is postponed months to years after the loss of a patient, especially a child. Initially, the family member may not be able to grieve appropriately, because of an inability to cope, or the pressing need to care for other family members.

Medical Errors

Assessment for patient safety must include a consideration of **medical errors**, unintentional but preventable mistakes in providing care. *Errors* are classified as failures to carry out a planned action or using the wrong plan, while an *adverse event* is the negative result of that error, such as an injury:

- Errors may result from commission (doing something) or omission (failing to do something).
- Errors can be active (resulting from contact between the patient and an aspect of the medical system, such as a nurse or piece of equipment).
- Errors can be latent, resulting from a failure of design in the system.
- Error chains are the series of events that lead to a negative outcome, usually identified through root cause analysis.
- Medical errors are most often identified after an adverse event occurs, but some may not be identified and are found on medical record reviews.

Safety Related to Medication Errors

There are about 7,000 deaths yearly in the United States attributed to medication errors. Studies indicate that there are errors in 1 in 5 doses of medication given to patients in hospitals. A caring environment is one in which patient safety is ensured with proper handling and administering of medications:

- Avoiding error-prone abbreviations or symbols. The Joint Commission has established a list of abbreviations to avoid, but mistakes are frequent with other abbreviations as well. In many cases, abbreviations and symbols should be avoided altogether or restricted to a limited approved list.
- Preventing errors from illegible handwriting. Handwritten orders should be block printed to reduce change of error.
- Instituting bar coding and scanners that allow the patient's wristband and medications to be scanned for verification.
- Providing lists of similarly named medications to educate staff.
- Establishing an institutional policy for administration of medications that includes protocols for verification of drug, dosage, and patient, as well as educating the patient about the medications.

Use of Restraints

Restraints are used to restrict movement, activity, and access. There are two primary types of restraints used with patients, clinical and behavioral. Behavioral restraints are more commonly used in the psychiatric unit or when patients are at risk of hurting themselves or others. More commonly, clinical restraints are used to ensure that the patient does not interfere with safe care. Restraints may be applied temporarily during a particular treatment or procedure or may be part of permanent care. The Joint Commission has issued strict guidelines for temporary restraints or those not part of standard care (such as postsurgical restraint):

- There must be a written policy.
- An assessment must be completed.
- An alternative method should be tried before applying a restraint.
- An order must be written.
- The least restrictive effective restraint should be used.
- A nurse must remove the restraint, assess, and document findings at least every 2 hours.

Staffing and Infection Control

Between 48,000 and 98,000 patients die each year in hospitals because of errors in patient safety. A caring environment must be a **safe environment** for children and their families. Patient safety is impacted by a number of factors:

- *Staffing practices*: Patient-staff ratios are of primary importance as studies have indicated that fewer staff and long hours result in more errors. This is especially true in acute/critical care units, or other specialized units. The expertise of the staff is another important factor. Studies indicate that increased proportion of care (in hours) by registered nurses decreases both hospital stay and complications.
- *Infection control*: The rates of hospital infections have steadily increased with pathogens (such as *Staphylococcus aureus* and *MRSA)* endemic in some institutions. Patients with invasive devices, such as central lines or ventilators, are at increased risk. Much infection is related to poor handwashing and infection control practices on the part of staff.

CDC Isolation Guidelines

Tier 1, Standard Precautions

Through the years, the CDC has issued a number of different guidelines for isolation precautions. The 1996 CDC isolation guidelines were an update from the Universal Precautions guidelines that dealt with blood and some body fluids but did not directly address other types of transmission. There are now two tiers of isolation precautions. Tier 1 deals with standard precautions that should be in place for all patients: *Standard precautions* include protection from all blood and body fluids and include the use of gloves, face barriers, and gowns as needed to avoid being splashed with fluids. Handwashing remains central to infection control and should be with plain (not antimicrobial) soap or instant antiseptic. Private rooms are used for those who contaminate the environment (e.g., uncontrolled diarrhea, cough) or are unhygienic. If no private room is available, patients with the same type of infection or same colonizing organism may share a room.

Tier 2, Transmission-Based Precautions, Airborne and Droplet

Tier 2 of the CDC isolation guidelines protects from three types of transmission. The first type provides protection from diseases spread by small airborne droplets (less than 5 mm), including measles, tuberculosis, and varicella.

- *Airborne precautions* include placing a patient in a private room with monitored negative airflow and the door closed. People who are susceptible to the disease, such as those not immunized against measles, should not enter the room. Respiratory precautions (a mask) should be worn if the patient has suspected or confirmed tuberculosis. Patient should wear mask outside of room.
- The second type provides protection from diseases spread by large airborne droplets (greater than 5 mm), easily spread by talking, coughing, or sneezing, but that do not travel more than 3 feet. Diseases include viral influenza, pertussis, streptococcal pharyngitis or pneumonia, *Neisseria meningitides*, and mumps.
- *Droplet precautions* include a private room. Staff and visitors who are within 3 feet of the patient must wear masks, and the patient must wear a mask outside of the room.

Tier 2, Transmission-Based Precautions, Contact

Tier 2 of the CDC isolation guidelines includes the third type, contact, which provides protection from diseases spread by direct hand-to-hand or skin-to-skin contact, such as those with significant infection or colonization and those who have suspected or confirmed multidrug resistance, which may include vancomycin-resistant *Enterococci* and *Staphylococcus aureus.*

- *Contact precautions* include placing the patient in a private room or room with someone with the same infection. Gloves should be used as for standard precautions but should immediately be removed and hands sanitized after contact with infective material. A clean protective gown should be worn inside the room for close contact with patient, including caring for a patient who is incontinent or has uncontained drainage. The patient should not leave the room if possible and equipment should be dedicated for patient use or disinfected before use by other patients.
- Some diseases may require some combination of airborne, droplet, and contact precautions: Lassa fever, Marburg virus, and smallpox.

Therapeutic Communication

Therapeutic communication begins with respect for the patient/family and the assumption that all communication, verbal and nonverbal, has meaning. Listening must be done empathetically. Techniques that facilitate communication include:

Introduction	Make a personal introduction and use the patient's name: "Mrs. Brown, I am Susan Williams, your nurse."
Encouragement	Use an open-ended opening statement: "Is there anything you'd like to discuss?"
	Acknowledge comments: "Yes," and "I understand."
	Allow silence and observe nonverbal behavior rather than trying to force conversation.
	Ask for clarification if statements are unclear.
	Reflect statements back (use sparingly): Patient: "I hate this hospital." Nurse: "You hate this hospital?"

Empathy	Make observations: "You are shaking," and "You seem worried."
	Recognize feelings: Patient: "I want to go home." Nurse: "It must be hard to be away from your home and family."
	Provide information as honestly and completely as possible about condition, treatment, and procedures, and respond to patient's questions and concerns.
Exploration	Verbally express implied messages: Patient: "This treatment is too much trouble." Nurse: "You think the treatment isn't helping you?"
	Explore a topic but allow the patient to terminate the discussion without further probing: "I'd like to hear how you feel about that."
Orientation	Indicate reality: Patient: "Someone is screaming." Nurse: "That sound was an ambulance siren."
	Comment on distortions without directly agreeing or disagreeing: Patient: "That nurse promised I didn't have to walk again." Nurse: "Really? That's surprising because the doctor ordered physical therapy twice a day."
Collaboration	Work together to achieve better results: "Maybe if we talk about this, we can figure out a way to make the treatment easier for you."
Validation	Seek validation: "Do you feel better now?" or "Did the medication help you breathe better?"

NONTHERAPEUTIC COMMUNICATION

While using therapeutic communication is important, it is equally important to avoid interjecting nontherapeutic communication, which can effectively block effective communication. *Avoid the following*:

- Meaningless clichés: "Don't worry. Everything will be fine." "Isn't it a nice day?"
- Providing advice: "You should..." or "The best thing to do is...." When patients ask for advice, it is better to provide facts and encourage the patient to reach a decision.
- Inappropriate approval that prevents the patient from expressing true feeling or concerns:
  - Patient: "I shouldn't cry about this."
  - Nurse: "That's right! You're an adult!"
- Asking for an explanation of behavior that is not directly related to patient care and requires analysis and explanation of feelings: "Why are you so upset?"
- Agreeing with rather than accepting and responding to patient's statements can make it difficult for the patient to change his/her statement or opinion later: "I agree with you," or "You are right."

Methods to promote a caring and supportive environment, avoiding nontherapeutic communication, include:

- Negative judgments: "You should stop arguing with the nurses."
- Devaluing patient's feelings: "Everyone gets upset at times."
- Disagreeing directly: "That can't be true," or "I think you are wrong."
- Defending against criticism: "The doctor is not being rude; he's just very busy today."
- Subject change to avoid dealing with uncomfortable topics:
  - Patient: "I'm never going to get well."
  - Nurse: "Your family will be here in just a few minutes."

- Inappropriate literal responses, even as a joke, especially if the patient is at all confused or having difficulty expressing ideas:
  - Patient: "There are bugs crawling under my skin."
  - Nurse: "I'll get some buy spray."
- Challenge to establish reality often just increases confusion and frustration: "If you were dying, you wouldn't be able to yell and kick!"

Complementary Therapies

Complementary therapies are used as well as conventional medical treatment and should be included if this is what the patient/family wants. This empowers the family to take some control. Complementary therapies vary widely and most can easily be incorporated into the plan of care. The National Center for Complementary and Alternative Medicine recognizes the following:

- Whole medical systems include medical systems, such as homeopathic, naturopathic medicine, acupuncture, and Chinese herbal medications.
- Mind-body medicine can include support groups, meditation, music, art, or dance therapy.
- Biologically based practices include the use of food, vitamins, or nutrition for healing.
- Manipulative/body-based programs include massage or other types of manipulation, such as chiropractic treatment.
- Energy therapies may be biofield therapies intended to affect the aura (energy field) that some believe surrounds all living things. These therapies include therapeutic touch and Reiki. Bioelectromagnetic-based therapies use a variety of magnetic fields.

Assisting the Caregiver

Caregivers for children are most often the parents and for elderly parents, the children, with the greatest burden of care often falling on the women. Caregiving can be extremely stressful, especially if the patient suffers from a chronic or serious disease. Part of caring practices is to recognize that the caregivers need care as well.

- *Conflict resolution* brings people with conflict together with a neutral person or group in order to attempt to negotiate or reach agreement. Nurses are in a unique position to assist with conflict resolution because they see people at their most vulnerable when they are dealing with stress.
- *Debriefing* allows the caregiver to talk about experiences that have caused trauma or stress.
- *Crisis intervention* takes place when an individual is overwhelmed by a situation and is not able to function adequately. It involves intervening during the crisis in order to help the person stabilize and to help him/her to function and to facilitate problem solving.

Communicating Complex Issues

The nursing environment is increasingly complex and must include meeting the needs of various members of the health care community and administration, as well as those of the patient/family. The nurse often stands at a central point between the patient/family on one side and other care providers and/or interested parties on the other. Especially in situations of severe illness, the patient/family often feel as though they are at the mercy of the health care community and are powerless. Because of this, the nurse must always represent the best interests of the patients/families and must interpret and communicate on their behalf so that there is consistency of care and consideration and understanding of their needs. It is important for the nurse to recognize that the patients/families are in a vulnerable position and need advocacy and caring to ensure that other caregivers respect their needs and preferences.

Caring Practices

Caring Practices

Caring practices encompass all nursing activities that respond to the individual patient's and family's needs in a caring, compassionate, and therapeutic environment to promote patient comfort and prevent unnecessary suffering. Caring practices recognize inner strength and its relation to healing, and seek to enhance the dignity of the individual through vigilance, nurturing, and skilled technical and basic nursing practices. Levels of caring practices include:

- Level 1: This nurse provides a safe environment and cares for the present basic needs of the patient without focus on future needs and considers death a potential outcome.
- Level 3: This nurse provides compassionate care, responding to changes in the patient, and acts of kindness, while accepting death as a possible outcome and providing measures to ensure good end-of-life care and a peaceful death.
- Level 5: This nurse is fully engaged in patient care and understands and interprets patient/family dynamics and needs, ensuring comfort, dignity, and safety while respecting the individual and family.

Standards of Advance Practice

The acute care nurse practitioner (ACNP) is guided by the standards of advance practice, which provide the framework for practice and describe the ACNP's responsibilities, related to the values and priorities of the profession:

- *Care process*: In assessing, diagnosing, developing, and implementing a plan of care, and evaluating the patient's response, the ACNP must use the scientific method and national standards as the basis for care.
- *Establishing priorities*: Providing education and encouraging the patient/family to take an active role in self care is of primary concern. The ACNP must ensure that the patient can make informed decisions. The ACNP must assist the patient through all aspects of health care to ensure patient safety and optimal care.
- *Collaboration*: The ACNP is a member of the interdisciplinary health team and consults with others when appropriate and refers the patient to specialists as needed. When collaboration is mandated by law, the ACNP complies with all requirements.
- *Documentation*: The ACNP keeps accurate, legal, legible records and maintains patient confidentiality. The ACNP ensures that the patient signs a release before providing medical records to other parties.
- *Patient advocacy*: The ACNP advocates for the individual patient in the process of care but also advocates for patients at the state and national level in order to facilitate patient access to care and improve the quality of care.
- *Continuous quality improvement*: The ACNP recognizes the need for constant learning, evaluation, and reevaluation, and participates in quality review, continuing education while maintaining certification and utilizing clinical guidelines and standards of care.
- *Research and education*: The ACNP initiates, participates in, and utilizes the results of research in clinical practice.

Professional Role and Policy

As part of the scope of practice, the nurse practitioner is able to provide and augment primary care to children/families through a number of different services:

- *Consultation* services may include a variety of services, such as assessing growth and development and risk factors, providing interventions, such as diet and exercise programs, and educating children/parents.

- *Referral services* include referring children to physicians, such as orthopedic specialists, and to organizations or agencies, such as drug rehabilitation programs.
- *Coordination services*, with the nurse maintaining contact and receiving reports from referrals in order to provide an integrated plan of care, serves as a valuable service to children/parents, who often must deal with many different health care providers who have little or no contact with each other. This type of service can prevent unnecessary duplications of service but also ensure that findings are not overlooked.

Both *prescribing* medications and treatment and ordering diagnostic tests are within the scope of practice of nurse practitioners, but as with other aspects of practice, each state establishes how that will be carried out. Additionally, insurance reimbursement varies from one area to another and must be considered:

- *Prescription*: Terminology varies from state to state with nurse practitioners allowed to "furnish" or "prescribe" some types of medications. In some states they may do so independently; in others, they must be "supervised" by a physician under whose auspices they provide care to patients. The nurse practitioner should maintain a list of medications and consider cost-effectiveness when ordering medications.
- *Diagnostics:* Nurse practitioners can order laboratory, ECG, and radiographic tests for routine screening and health assessment as well as diagnosis based on assessment. There are limitations, depending upon the individual state nursing practice act.

Promoting Caring Environment

Promoting a caring and supportive environment means ensuring that the patient is comfortable. According to Joint Commission guidelines and federal law, all patients have to right to pain management, and this applies to infants and children. It is not enough to recognize this; procedures must be in place to ensure that all staff are committed to reducing pain and that patients/families be apprised of the right and benefits of pain management. There are steps that the institution can take in this process:

- Create an interdisciplinary team to research, provide guidelines, and communicate goals.
- Assess pain management procedures already in place to determine effectiveness or need for change.
- Establish a minimum standard that should be legally followed.
- Clarify responsibility for pain control and imbed this in the standards of practice.
- Provide information about pain control to all levels of care providers.
- Educate patients to understand they are entitled to rapid response.
- Educate staff to institutionalize pain management.

The Pain Scale

Pain is subjective and may be influenced by the individual's pain threshold (the smallest stimulus that produces the sensation of pain) and pain tolerance (the maximum degree of pain that a person can tolerate). The most common current pain assessment tool for preteens/adolescents is the 1 to 10 scale:

- 0 = no pain
- 1 to 2 = mild pain
- 3 to 5 = moderate pain
- 6 to 7 = severe pain
- 8 to 9 = very severe pain
- 10 = excruciating pain.

However, there is more to pain assessment than a number on a scale. Assessment includes information about onset, duration, and intensity. Identifying what triggers pain and what relieves it can be very useful when developing a plan for pain management. Patients may show very different behavior when they are in pain:

Some may cry and moan with minor pain, and others may exhibit little difference in behavior when truly suffering. Thus, judging pain by behavior can lead to the wrong conclusions.

Patients with cognitive impairment or inability to verbalize pain may not be able to indicate the degree of pain, even by using a face scale with pictures of smiling to crying faces. The Pain Assessment in Advanced Dementia (PAINAD) scale may be helpful, especially for those with Alzheimer disease. Careful observation of nonverbal behavior can indicate that the patient is in pain:

- *Respirations*: Patients often have more rapid and labored breathing as pain increases, with short periods of hyperventilation or Cheyne-Stokes respirations.
- *Vocalization*: Patients may remain negative in speech or speak quietly and reluctantly. They may moan or groan. As pain increases, they may call out, moan or groan loudly, or cry.
- *Facial expression*: Patients may appear sad or frightened, may frown or grimace, especially on activities that increase pain.
- *Body language*: Patients may be tense, fidgeting, or pacing, and as pain increases may become rigid, clench fists, or lie in fetal position. They may become increasingly combative.
- *Consolability*: Patients are less distractible or consolable with increased pain.

Collaboration

COLLABORATION

Collaboration is a team approach of working with a variety of others (physicians, nurses, dietitians, therapist, families, social workers, community leaders and members, clergy, intra- and interdisciplinary teams) in a cooperative manner, using good therapeutic communication skills, to ensure that each person is contributing optimally toward reaching patient goals and positive outcomes. Collaboration requires mutual respect, professional maturity, common purpose, and a positive sense of self. Levels of collaboration include:

- Level 1: This nurse participates in collaborative activities, learns from others, including mentors, and respects the input of others.
- Level 3: This nurse not only participates in collaborative activities but also initiates them and actively seeks learning opportunities.
- Level 5: This nurse takes a leadership role in collaborative activities by mentoring and teaching others while still seeking learning opportunities, and actively seeks additional resources as needed.

Nurses must learn the set of skills needed for collaboration in order to move nursing forward. Nurses must take an active role in gathering data for evidence-based practice to support nursing's role in health care and must share this information with other nurses and health care providers in order to plan staffing levels and to provide optimal care to patients. Increased and adequate staffing has consistently been shown to reduce adverse outcomes, but there is a well-documented shortage of nurses in the United States, and more than half of current RNs work outside the hospital. Increased patient loads not only increase adverse outcomes but also increase job dissatisfaction and burnout. In order to manage the challenges facing nursing, nurses must develop skills needed for collaboration:

- Be willing to compromise.
- Communicate clearly. Specific challenges and problems.
- Focus on the task.
- Work with teams.

INVOLVEMENT WITH EXTERNAL AGENCIES

The acute care nurse must initiate and facilitate involvement with external agencies because many have direct impacts on patient care and needs:

- Industry can include other facilities sharing interests in patient care or pharmaceutical companies. It is important for nursing to have a dialogue with drug companies about their products and how they are used in the pediatric/geriatric populations because many medications are prescribed to children and older adults without validating studies for dose or efficacy.
- Payors have a vested interest in containing health care costs, so providing information and representing the interests of the patient is important.
- Community groups may provide resources for patients and families, both in terms of information and financial or other assistance.
- Political agencies are increasingly important as new laws are considered about nurse-patient ratios and infection control in many states.
- Public health agencies are partners in health care with other facilities and must be included, especially in issues related to communicable disease.

Assisting others to understand and use resources and expertise of others requires a commitment in terms of time and effort:

- Coaching others on methods of collaboration can include providing information in the form of handouts about effective communication strategies and, in turn, modeling this type of communication with the staff being coached.
- Team meetings are commonly held on nursing units and provide an opportunity to model collaboration and suggest the need for outside expertise to help with planning patient care plans. The mentoring nurse can initiate discussions about resources that are available in the facility or the community.
- Selecting a diverse group for teams or inviting those with expertise in various areas to join the team when needed can help team members to appreciate and understand how to use the input of other resources.

Nurse-Physician and Nurse-Nurse Collaboration

Traditionally, the nurse worked under the authority of the physician, but with specialization and advanced practice and increases in the complexity of medical care, the roles of nurse and physician have become much more collaborative, with each functioning within their scope of practice. The nurse and physician often collaborate and cooperate in diagnosing and planning treatment. To add to the complexity, staff nurses, such as acute care nurses, may also collaborate in a similar manner with nurse specialists or nurse practitioners, who often accompany physicians on rounds while staff nurses are too busy to take time for rounds. The nurse practitioner is usually on the ward for much longer periods of time than the physician, facilitating collaboration with other nurses. Direct contact is an important element in collaboration. In order for nurse-physician collaboration to be successful, methods must be employed to improve contact and communication.

Collaboration with Families

One of the most important forms of collaboration is that between the nurse and the patient/family, but this type of collaboration is often overlooked. Nurses and others in the health care team must always remember that the point of collaborating is to improve patient care, and this means that the patient and patient's family must remain central to all planning. For example, including family in planning for a patient takes time initially, but sitting down and asking the patient and family, "What do you want?" and using the synergy model to evaluate patient's (and family's) characteristics can provide valuable information. This can save time in the long run and facilitate planning and expenditure of resources. Families, and even young children, often want to participate in care and planning and feel validated and more positive toward the medical system when they are included.

Staffing Needs

As nursing resources become more limited, staffing must be done efficiently to best meet the needs of patients. The synergy model can be used in a collaborative effort to identify those patients who are most in need of care. This requires observation and evidence-based research. Often, different units use different criteria to determine staffing needs, but the synergy model can be used across disciplines and in different types of units. For example, one hospital used to synergy model to determine which patients required a 1:1 patient-staff ratio in the critical care unit. When considering the patient characteristics (resiliency, vulnerability, stability, complexity, resource availability, participation in care, participation in decision making, and predictability), staff determined that 4 characteristics (stability, complexity, vulnerability, and resiliency) at level 1 could be used as the determinant for 1:1 twenty-four-hour care. Those at levels 2 and 3 required fewer hours of 1:1 care so that the nurse could also care for other patients.

COMMUNICATION SKILLS NECESSARY FOR COLLABORATION

Collaboration requires a number of communication skills that differ from those involved in communication between nurse and patient. These skills include:

- *Using an assertive approach*: It is important for the nurse to honestly express opinions and to state them clearly and with confidence, but the nurse must do so in a calm, nonthreatening manner.
- *Making casual conversation*: It is easier to communicate with people with whom one has a personal connection. Asking open-ended questions, asking about other's work, or commenting on someone's contributions helps to establish a relationship. The time before meetings, during breaks, and after meetings presents an opportunity for this type of conversation.
- *Being competent in public speaking*: Collaboration requires that a nurse be comfortable speaking and presenting ideas to groups of people, and doing so helps the person to gain credibility. This is a skill that must be practiced.
- *Communicating in writing*: The written word remains a critical component of communication, and the nurse should be able to communicate clearly and grammatically.

DELEGATION OF TASKS

The scope of nursing practice includes delegation of tasks to unlicensed assistive personnel, provided those personnel have adequate training and knowledge to carry out the tasks. Delegation should be used to manage the workload and to provide adequate and safe care. The nurse who delegates remains accountable for patient outcomes and for supervision of the person to whom the task was delegated, so the nurse must consider the following:

- whether knowledge, skills, and training of the unlicensed assistive personnel provides the ability to perform the delegated task
- whether the patient's condition and needs have been properly evaluated and assessed
- whether the nurse is able to provide ongoing supervision.

Delegation should be done in a manner that reduces liability by providing adequate communication. This includes specific directions about the task, including what needs to be done, when, and for how long. Expectations related to consultation, reporting, and completion of tasks should be clearly defined. The nurse should be available to assist if necessary.

On major responsibility of leadership and management in performance improvement teams is using delegation effectively. The purpose of having a team is so that the work is shared, and leaders can cripple themselves by taking on too much of the workload. Additionally, failure to delegate shows an inherent distrust in team members. Delegation includes:

- Assessing the skills and available time of the team members, and determining if a task is suitable for an individual.
- Assigning tasks, with clear instructions that include explanation of objectives and expectations, including a timeline.
- Ensuring that the tasks are completed properly and on time by monitoring progress but not micromanaging.
- Reviewing the final results and recording outcomes.

Because the leader is ultimately responsible for the delegated work, mentoring, monitoring, and providing feedback and intervention as necessary during this process is a necessary component of leadership. While delegated tasks may not always be completed successfully, they represent an opportunity for learning.

Common Vision of Care

Facilitating the creation of a common vision for care within the health care system begins with the organization/facility working collaboratively to create teams and an organization focused on serving the patient/family. A common vision should be the ideal in any organization, but achieving such a goal requires a true collaborative effort:

- Inclusion of all levels of staff across the organization/facility, both those in nursing and non-nursing positions.
- Consensus building through discussions, inservice, and team meetings to bring about convergence of diverse viewpoints.
- Facilitation that values creativity and provides encouragement during the process.
- Vision statement incorporating the common vision that is accessible to all staff.
- Recognition that a common vision is an organic concept that may evolve over time and should be reevaluated regularly and changed as needed to reflect the needs of the organization, patients, families, and staff.

Team Building

Leading, facilitating, and participating in performance improvement teams requires a thorough understanding of the dynamics of team building:

- *Initial interactions*: This is the time when members begin to define their roles and develop relationships, determining if they are comfortable in the group.
- *Power issues*: The members observe the leader and determine who controls the meeting and how control is exercised, beginning to form alliances.
- *Organizing*: Methods to achieve work are clarified and team members begin to work together, gaining respect for each other's contributions and working toward a common goal.
- *Team identification*: Interactions often become less formal as members develop rapport, and members are more willing to help and support each other to achieve goals.
- *Excellence*: This develops through a combination of good leadership, committed team members, clear goals, high standards, external recognition, spirit of collaboration, and a shared commitment to the process.

Team Contracts

Many of the problems that arise in team processes could be avoided if the team members reached consensus about expectations of working within the group. One method is to complete a team contract at an initial meeting with all members participating. Team contracts include sections on the following:

- *Roles*: The specific responsibility of each member of the team, including the leader, should be delineated.
- *Discussion:* The manner in which discussion is to be held (agenda driven, Robert's Rules of Order, open discussion) should be outlined.
- *Time*: The amount of time that members are expected to commit to team activities should be stated, including time for meetings.
- *Conduct*: Acceptable parameters for behavior should be clarified, including those for the individual and the group.
- *Conflict resolution*: Triggers for conflict resolution and methods should be agreed upon.
- *Reports*: The types of reports, timeline, and responsibility for preparing the reports must be clear.
- *Consequences*: Failure to follow the contract should result in consequences that are clearly identified.

TEAM MEETINGS

Leading and facilitating improvement teams requires utilizing good techniques for meetings. Considerations include:

- *Scheduling*: Both the time and the place must be convenient and conducive to working together, so the leader must review the work schedules of those involved, finding the most convenient time. Venues or meeting rooms should allow for sitting in a circle or around a table to facilitate equal exchange of ideas. Any necessary technology, such as computers or overhead projectors, or other equipment, such as white boards, should be available.
- *Preparation*: The leader should prepare a detailed agenda that includes a list of items for discussion.
- *Conduction*: Each item of the agenda should be discussed, soliciting input from all group members. Tasks should be assigned to individual members based on their interest and part in the process in preparation for the next meeting. The leader should summarize input and begin a tentative future agenda.
- *Observation*: The leader should observe the interactions, including verbal and nonverbal communication, and respond to these.

TEAM STRUCTURE

The appropriate team structure is very important in performance improvement because creating a team does not in itself ensure teamwork. The team must be comprised of individuals whose skills complement each other and who have a shared purpose because outcomes will depend on the collaborative efforts of the group rather than individuals within the group. Accordingly, the collective team is accountable for outcomes rather than individuals. When creating teams, the team structure, important elements must be considered:

- *Size*: Teams of fewer than 10 members are most effective.
- *Skills*: Team members should have complementary skills that encompass technical, problem solving, decision making, and interpersonal.
- *Performance goals*: Teams should be allowed a degree of autonomy in producing action plans for performance improvement, based on strategic goals and objectives.
- *Unified approach*: The teams should be created according to the model of performance improvement, but should have some flexibility in working together.
- *Accountability*: The team members are collectively accountable rather than individually.

CROSS-FUNCTIONAL TEAMS

Cross-functional teams (also referred to as interdisciplinary) comprise individuals from various skill levels or disciplines who work together to accomplish one or more functions. In some cases, cross-functional teams may be *ad hoc,* operating for a short time to accomplish specific goals, but other times they become a permanent part of performance improvement. Cross-functional teams are most useful when dealing with problems or performance activities that cross disciplines, especially if a broad range of expertise and skills is needed. Selecting team members with the correct mix of abilities is important for success. The roles for the team members should be clearly outlined, as well as expected outcomes. Adequate training must be provided to assist cross-functional team members in working together as a unit.

Cross-functional teams are particularly useful in the following:

- developing new processes
- implementing organization-wide performance changes or technology
- controlling costs and increasing cost-benefit ratio.

SELF-DIRECTED WORK TEAMS

Self-directed work teams are groups of individuals working together to achieve a common goal, such as improving a process or producing a product. While the members may be trained cross-functionally, they usually have individual functions within the group. Usually, the teams have an assigned task or tasks for which they are accountable but have the authority to manage the functions on their own and make decisions without the direction of administration. As with other types of teams, self-directed work teams may be *ad hoc* or permanent and the degree of autonomy may vary from one organization to another. Self-directed work teams may do the following:

- Plan and establish priorities.
- Organize and manage budget.
- Manage work schedules and assignments.
- Engage in problem-solving activities and make corrections.
- Monitor and evaluate performance.
- Coordinate with other teams or individuals.
- Chose or hire team members.

Interdisciplinary Collaboration

Interdisciplinary collaboration is absolutely critical to nursing practice if the needs and best interests of the patients and families are central. Interdisciplinary practice begins with the nurse and physician but extends to pharmacists, social workers, occupational and physical therapists, nutritionists, and a wide range of allied health care providers, all of whom cooperate in diagnosis and treatment. State regulations determine to some degree how much autonomy a nurse can have in diagnosing and treating. While nurses have increasingly gained more legal rights, they have also become more dependent upon collaboration with others for their expertise and for referrals if the patient's needs extend beyond the nurse's ability to provide assistance. Additionally, the prescriptive ability of nurses varies from state to state, with some requiring direct supervision by other disciplines (such as physicians), while others require particular types of supervisory arrangements, depending upon the circumstances and nurse's certification.

Intra- and Interdisciplinary Teams

The complexity of patient care requires collaboration among intra- and interdisciplinary teams. Often the nurse is in the position to evaluate problems that arise, to seek collaboration, and to recognize when multiple perspectives can be helpful in solving conflicts or making decisions about health care. The nurse can facilitate creation of teams for problem solving. Collaboration requires open sharing of ideas and respect for the expertise of the individual. Collaboration requires more than just talking, however. In many cases it may be more formalized, with specialized committees formed in order to solve specific problems. Studies have indicated that patients benefit from collaborative efforts between nurse and physician, and this benefit extends to others as well. In a collaborative environment, all of the participants benefit from sharing ideas and discussion that can lead to innovative problem solving.

There are a number of skills that are needed to lead and facilitate coordination of intra- and interdisciplinary teams:

- Communicating openly is essential with all members encouraged to participate as valued members of a cooperative team.
- Avoiding interrupting or interpreting the point another is trying to make allows free flow of ideas.
- Avoiding jumping to conclusions, which can effectively shut off communication.
- Active listening requires paying attention and asking questions for clarification rather than challenging others' ideas.
- Respecting others' opinions and ideas, even when opposed to one's own, is absolutely essential.
- Reacting and responding to facts rather than feelings allows one to avoid angry confrontations or diffuse anger.
- Clarifying information or opinions stated can help avoid misunderstandings.
- Keeping unsolicited advice out of the conversation shows respect for others and allows them to solicit advice without feeling pressured.

Professional Leadership and Accountability

Nurses, especially those in leadership positions, have a responsibility to assist others with professional leadership and accountability within the health care team and community. Collaboration needs an ongoing commitment that includes mentoring, coaching, and teaching others. Nursing must be involved in the following:

- Making decisions at all levels of an organization/facility.
- Taking an active role in strategic planning.
- Assuming responsibility for standards of nursing care.
- Assessing and selecting equipment and supplies as well as electronic equipment, including information systems.
- Assisting in planning for utilization of resources.
- Analyzing all decisions with respect to patient outcomes.
- Supporting staff education and development, including training for management positions and opportunities to acquire continuing education hours.
- Facilitating access to research and both internal and external resources.
- Allowing staff members time to consider their place in the organization and their own practice.

Leadership Values and Commitment

Leadership must be consistent. It succeeds by providing staff with direction and guidance that shows by example, and explaining why things need to be done rather than directing how this must be achieved. A good leader fosters values by focusing on the right way to do things rather than on errors or poor performance. By engaging staff in all part of the processes, a leader engenders a sense of commitment and collaboration on the part of the staff. This commitment cannot be achieved through rules, regulation, threats, and criticism. A good leader must demonstrate integrity, welcome diversity, be open-minded, and search for competence. While a leader must have a thorough understanding of the organization/facility and its work, he or she must be able to look holistically. The leader must motivate others by providing structure and order, and have the ability to make decisions while continuing to learn and teach in order to create positive change.

Leadership must understand **motivation** because a positive perception of leadership motivates people to produce and improve performance. In order to understand what motivates staff members, the leader must set aside preconceived ideas and listen carefully, discovering the strengths of the individuals and groups within the organization or facility, and providing positive reinforcement and rewards. Leadership involves expecting excellence and removing barriers to employee involvement in the process so that employees feel empowered, recognized, and acknowledged as valuable. The responses of leadership should be based on actual assessment rather than preconceived ideas or biases. Studies have shown that the four things that motivate employees the most include:

- *Autonomy*: Allowing people to use their ideas.
- *Salary*: Providing adequate compensation for work done.
- *Recognition*: Appreciating the efforts that employees put forth.
- *Respect*: Listening to ideas.

Leadership Styles

Leadership styles often influence the perception of leadership values and commitment to collaboration. There are a number of different leadership styles:

- *Charismatic*: Depends upon personal charisma to influence people, and may be very persuasive, but this type leader may engage "followers" and relate to one group rather than the organization at large, limiting effectiveness.

- *Bureaucratic*: Follows organization rules exactly and expects everyone else to do so. This is most effective in handling cash flow or managing work in dangerous work environments. This type of leadership may engender respect but may not be conducive to change.
- *Autocratic*: Makes decisions independently and strictly enforces rules, but team members often feel left out of process and may not be supportive. This type of leadership is most effective in crisis situations, but may have difficulty gaining commitment of staff.
- *Consultative*: Presents a decision and welcomes input and questions although decisions rarely change. This type of leadership is most effective when gaining the support of staff is critical to the success of proposed changes.

Different leadership styles in developing leadership values and commitment to collaboration include:

- *Participatory*: Presents a potential decision and then makes the final decision based on input from staff or teams. This type of leadership is time-consuming and may result in compromises that are not wholly satisfactory to management or staff, but this process is motivating to staff who feel their expertise is valued.
- *Democratic*: Presents a problem and asks staff or teams to arrive at a solution, although the leader usually makes the final decision. This type of leadership may delay decision making, but staff and teams are often more committed to the solutions because of their input.
- *Laissez-faire* (free rein): Exerts little direct control but allows employees/ teams to make decisions with little interference. This may be effective leadership if teams are highly skilled and motivated, but in many cases this type of leadership is the product of poor management skills and little is accomplished because of this lack of leadership.

Resistance to Organizational Change

Performance improvement processes cannot occur without organizational change, and resistance to change is common for many people, so coordinating collaborative processes requires anticipating resistance and taking steps to achieve cooperation. Resistance often relates to concerns about job loss, increased responsibilities, and general denial or lack of understanding and frustration. Leaders can prepare others involved in the process of change by taking these steps:

- Be honest, informative, and tactful, giving people thorough information about anticipated changes and how the changes will affect them, including positives.
- Be patient in allowing people the time they need to contemplate changes and express anger or disagreement.
- Be empathetic in listening carefully to the concerns of others.
- Encourage participation, allowing staff to propose methods of implementing change, so they feel some sense of ownership.
- Establish a climate in which all staff members are encouraged to identify the need for change on an ongoing basis.
- Present further ideas for change to management.

Conflict Resolution

Conflict is an almost inevitable product of teamwork, and the leader must assume responsibility for conflict resolution. While conflicts can be disruptive, they can produce positive outcomes by forcing team members to listen to different perspectives and opening dialogue. The team should make a plan for dealing with conflict resolution. The best time for conflict resolution is when differences emerge but before open conflict and hardening of positions occur. The leader must pay close attention to the people and problems involved, listen carefully, and reassure those involved that their points of view are understood. Steps to conflict resolution include:

- Allow both sides to present their side of conflict without bias, maintaining a focus on opinions rather than individuals.
- Encourage cooperation through negotiation and compromise.
- Maintain the focus, providing guidance to keep the discussions on track and avoid arguments.
- Evaluate the need for renegotiation, formal resolution process, or third party.
- Utilize humor and empathy to diffuse escalating tensions.
- Summarize the issues, outlining key arguments.
- Avoid forcing resolution if possible

Systems Thinking

Facilitating Change

Facilitating change within a health care organization requires the creation of a common vision for care and begins with the organization/facility working collaboratively to create teams and an organization focused on serving the customers. A common vision should be the ideal in any organization, but achieving such a goal requires a true collaborative effort:

- Inclusion of all levels of staff across the organization/facility, both those in nursing and non-nursing positions.
- Consensus building through discussions, inservice, and team meetings to bring about convergence of diverse viewpoints.
- Facilitation that values creativity and provides encouragement during the process.
- Vision statement incorporating the common vision that is accessible to all staff.
- Recognition that a common vision is an organic concept that may evolve over time and should be reevaluated regularly and changed as needed to reflect the needs of the organization, patients, families, and staff.

Patient Care Practices

Patient care practices are established as part of the organizational structure:

- *The organizational mission* should be included in a mission statement that identifies the program and its function, and outlines in clear detail the purpose and strategy of the program. It is important for the organizational mission to be holistic, including the mission of the organization as a whole, with all parts represented. The mission statement is often followed by lists of committees and specific tasks, and their relationship to the organizational mission should be clarified.
- *Goals* should be achievable and are essentially outcomes that are expected of the organization. Objectives, then, are the measurable steps that must be taken to achieve the goals, and it is this level that directly impacts patient care practices. Each goal may have a number of objectives, and objectives may vary across the organizational structure in order for the system as a whole to accomplish a goal, in accordance with the mission.

Systems Thinking

Systems thinking is having the background knowledge and practical tools to manage both environmental and system resources, within and outside of the health care system, in order to solve problems for the patient/family and meet their needs. Solving problems requires a holistic view of the interrelationships and understanding of how structures, patterns, and events affect outcomes. Levels of systems thinking includes:

- Level 1: This nurse views himself/herself as the primary resource to meet the needs of the patient within the confines of the unit and does not recognize the need to negotiate.
- Level 3: This nurse looks beyond the unit and personal contributions to view the patient's progress through the entire system and sees the need to negotiate with others to provide the best resources available. However, he/she may lack the skills needed to do so.
- Level 5: This nurse is expert at understanding the organization holistically and uses a number of different strategies to negotiate with others and assist the patient with progress through the system.

Barriers to Systems Thinking

Barriers to system thinking can arise with the individual, the department, or the administrative level:

- *Identification with role rather than purpose*: People see themselves from the perspective of their role in the system, as nurse or physician, and are not able to step outside their preconceived ideas to view situations holistically or to accept the roles of others. They may lack the ability to look at situations as human beings first and professionals second.
- *Feelings of victimization*: People may blame the organization or the leadership for personal shortcomings or feel that there is nothing that they can do to improve or change situations. A feeling of victimization may permeate an institution to the point that meaningful communication cannot take place, and people are not open to change.
- *Relying on past experience*: New directions require new solutions, so being mired in the past or relying solely on past experience can prevent progress.
- *Autocratic views*: Some feel that their perceptions and practices are the only ones that are acceptable and often have a narrow focus so that they cannot view the system as a whole but focus on short-term outcomes. They fail to see that there are many aspects to a problem, affecting many parts of the system.
- *Failure to adapt*: Change is difficult for many individuals and institutions, but the medical world is changing rapidly, and this requires adaptability. Those who fail to adapt may feel threatened by changes and unsure of their ability to relearn new concepts, principles, and procedures.
- *Weak consensus*: Groups that arrive at easy or weak consensus without delving into important issues may delude themselves into believing that they have solved problems that remain concerns.

Delivery of Care

The delivery of care is impacted by a numerous forces:

- *Social forces* are increasing demand for access to treatment and medical services, both traditional and complementary. As society views equitable medical care as a right, then delivery of care must be available to all.
- *Political forces* affect medical care as the federal and state governments increasingly become purchasers of medical care, imposing their guidelines and limitations on the medical system.
- *Regulatory forces* may be local, state, or federal, and can have a profound effect on delivery of care and services, differing from one state or region to another.
- *Economic forces*, such as managed care or cost-containment committees, try to contain costs to insurers and facilities by controlling access to and duration of treatment, and limiting products. Economic pressure is working to prevent duplication of services in a geographical area, and providers are creating networks to purchase supplies and equipment directly.

Star Model

Innovative systems thinking and resource use among the health care team requires empowering staff to make decisions and to identify needs that require resource allocations. Administration needs to look for nursing leaders who are open to nontraditional methods and not afraid to change. One model to consider is the Star Model, based on a star diagram with strategy, structure, human resources, incentives, and information and decision making as the points around a core of systemic culture and values:

- Staff laziness or inability is rarely the root cause of systemic problems.
- There is more than one optimal system, depending on internal and external factors.
- One point is not more important than another.
- A change in one area usually necessitates a change in another.
- The culture and values cannot be changed directly but only indirectly through action on one of the points.
- Ingrained cultures and values can impede progress.

Concepts of Systems Thinking

The promotion of organizational values and commitment requires that the organization embody systems thinking and the associated concepts. Systems thinking focuses on how systems interrelate, with each part affecting the entire system. Concepts include:

- *Individual responsibility*: Individuals are encouraged to establish their own goals within the organization and to work toward a purpose.
- *Learning process*: The internalized beliefs of the staff are respected while building upon these beliefs to establish a mindset based on continuous learning and improvement.
- *Vision*: A sharing of organizational vision helps staff to understand the purpose of change and builds commitment.
- *Team process*: Teams are assisted to develop good listening and collaborative skills so that there is an increase in dialogue and an ability to reach consensus.
- *Systems thinking*: Staff members are encouraged to understand the interrelationship of all members of the organization and to appreciate how any change affects the whole.

Steps to Systems Thinking

- An approach to systems thinking is especially valuable in organizations in which there is lack of consensus, effective change is stalemated, and standards are inconsistent. Systems thinking is a critical thinking approach to problem solving that takes an organization-wide perspective. Steps include:
- T*he issue*: Describe the problem in detail without judgment or solutions.
- B*ehavior patterns*: This includes listing factors related to the problem, using graphs to outline possible trends.
- *Establish cause-effect relationships*: This may include using the Five Whys or other root cause analysis or feedback loops.
- P*atterns of performance/behavior*: Determine how variables affect outcomes and the types of patterns of behavior currently taking place.
- *Find solutions*: Discuss possible solutions and outcomes.
- *Institute performance-improvement activities*: Make changes and then monitor for changes in behavior.

Using Knowledge of System to Work with Internal and External Clients

A thorough understanding of the interrelatedness of all aspects of the system is necessary in working with internal and external clients:

- *Internal clients*: Those with direct responsibility for providing care to patients include nurses, physicians, various therapists, as well as administrative and support staff. Each has a role within the system to deliver care, but not one can function alone. The doctor is dependent upon nurses to provide treatment and care for the patient. The nurses in turn are dependent on others, such as laboratory staff, nutritional services, housekeeping, and physical therapists, to provide specialized services. All are dependent on administration to provide a working environment. Each must be considered.
- *External clients*: Those that provide services but not direct patient care may include sales representatives for pharmaceutical or medical equipment companies, regulatory agencies, or other institutions, such as extended care facilities. All provide services that can impact the system.

Strategies to Optimize Outcomes

Optimal outcomes can be achieved when the characteristics of the patient and the nurse competencies match within the framework of an interrelated system in which the patient/family is an equal partner. Outcomes are derived from different components:

- *Patient*: Trust in the health care provider based on perceived caring and competency is an essential outcome and links with the functional ability of the patient and the quality of life. Patients/families must feel satisfied with care.
- *Nurse*: Measurable outcomes are associated with nursing and include physiological changes, occurrence or prevention of infection, and effectiveness of nursing care and treatments. The nurse serves to coordinate many aspects of care relating to outcomes.
- *System*: Outcomes relate to the delivery of care that is consistently both high quality and cost-effective. This includes data regarding rates of re-hospitalization, length of hospitalization, and optimal utilization of resources linked to cost data.

Integration of Key Concepts

There are a number of key concepts related to quality that must be communicated to all members of an organization through inservice, workshops, newsletters, fact sheets, and team meetings. Quality care/performance should be:

- *Appropriate* to needs and in keeping with best practices.
- *Accessible* to the individual despite financial, cultural, or other barriers.
- *Competent* with practitioners who are well-trained and adhering to standards.
- *Coordinated* among all health care providers.
- *Effective* in achieving outcomes based on the current state of knowledge.
- *Efficient* in methods of achieving the desired outcomes.
- *Preventive*, allowing for early detection and prevention of problems.
- *Respectful* and caring with consideration of the individual needs given primary importance.
- *Safe* so that the organization is free of hazards or dangers that may put patients or others at risk.

Performance Improvement

All members of an organization should be provided access to performance improvement information with which they are involved, with management ensuring that confidentiality is maintained so that identifiers of patients and practitioners are removed from the data. Peer review activities must follow state regulations, and these records may be maintained separately from those disseminated. Reports are often provided to management at meetings, and then management disseminates them to other staff through staff meetings. Reports are presented to upper levels of management and the governing board on a regularly scheduled basis, often quarterly with annual summary reports. Feedback on performance measure should be given to teams, departments, and leaders. Organizations may use newsletters, e-mail, or the Internet to post performance information, but all methods should include contact information for those who wish to comment or ask questions in order to encourage organization-wide participation.

Organizational Transparency

Organizational transparency is a fairly new concept for the health care industry, which has been better known for concealment of data. There is much pressure from the public to make health care organizations more transparent as evidence about unnecessary surgery, costs, infection rates, and other negative information have been made public. The organization must be committed to transparency of pricing and quality so that both staff and patients have realistic expectations and understanding. Information that should be available includes:

- *Financial information*: Costs and profit information should be available.
- *Performance measures*: The factors that are valued and measured should be clearly outlined.
- *Outcomes*: Both positive (improvements) and negatives (failure to improve) should be presented to demonstrate quality.
- *Safety records*: Information about safety concerns must be disseminated.
- *Medical records*: These should be open to the individual patients.
- *Leadership qualities/promotion*: There should be clear understanding of parameters for promotion and leadership.

Different Perspectives

Systems thinking can be a challenge because people look at the needs and goals of an organization from very different perspectives. While those involved in direct patient care, such as nurses and physicians, may be most concerned with improving patient outcomes, those with other responsibilities, such as financial affairs or human resources, may envision a different path toward achieving these outcomes or may be concerned with other outcomes. For example, the financial affairs representative's goal may be to decrease expenditures while the human resources representative wants to reduce absenteeism. The challenge then is not to fight for the most important concern but to try to find a solution that addresses all concerns. In this case, more effective staffing can reduce expenditures while improving patient care and reducing stress and burnout, resulting in a decrease in absenteeism—which in turn reduces expenditures and improves patient care. Thus, an effective solution perpetuates positive outcomes.

Clinical Inquiry

Clinical inquiry is a continual process of questioning and evaluating practice in order to provide innovative and outstanding care through application of the results of research and experience. Clinical inquiry requires a desire to acquire new knowledge, openness to accepting advice from mentors and other health and allied professionals, competency in identifying clinical problems, and the ability search the literature for research, critical skills to interpret research findings, and a willingness and ability to design and participate in research. Levels of clinical inquiry include:

- Level 1: This nurse recognizes problems and seeks advice, follows industry standards and guidelines, and seeks further knowledge.
- Level 3: This nurse questions industry standards and guidelines as well as current practice and utilizes research and education to improve patient care.
- Level 5: This nurse is able to deviate from industry standards and guidelines when necessary for the individual patient and utilizes literature review and clinical research to gain knowledge, establish new practices, and improve patient care.

Evidence-Based Practice Guidelines

Evidence-based practice guidelines for such things as standing medicine orders or antibiotic protocols are in common use, but decisions are often made based on studies that lack internal and/or external validity or on expert opinion colored by personal bias, so the process of establishing evidence-based practice guidelines should be done systematically. Including those who are resistive to the process often helps to facilitate the establishment of guidelines, but it is important that decisions be made on solid evidence as much as possible. Simply dispensing evidence-based practice guidelines often does not change practice, so consideration must be given to implementation. Decisions must be made as to whether the use of the guidelines is mandatory as standing orders and to what degree individual practitioners can choose other options. Guidelines that are too rigid may be counterproductive. In some case, establishing guidelines may affect cost-reimbursement from third-party payers.

Steps to Evidence-Based Practice Guidelines Include:

- *Focus on the topic/methodology*: This includes outlining possible interventions/treatments for review, choosing patient populations and settings, and determining significant outcomes. Search boundaries (such as types of journals, types of studies, dates of studies) should be determined.
- *Evidence review*: This includes review of literature, critical analysis of studies, and summarizing of results, including pooled meta-analysis.
- *Expert judgment*: Recommendations based on personal experience from a number of experts may be utilized, especially if there is inadequate evidence based on review, but this subjective evidence should be explicated and acknowledged.
- *Policy considerations*: This includes cost-effectiveness, access to care, insurance coverage, availability of qualified staff, and legal implications.
- *Policy*: A written policy must be completed with recommendations. Common practice is to utilize letter guidelines, with "A" the most highly recommended, usually based the quality of supporting evidence.
- *Review*: The completed policy should be submitted to peers for review and comments before instituting the policy.

Selection of Outcomes Measures

Because both process and outcomes are equally important in performance improvement, consider whether the focus is to be on the process or the outcome. Both a short-term and long-term focuses for outcomes should be established. Short-term outcomes show results directly related to the process, allowing for modifications/interventions of the process. Long-term outcomes, however, often relate more to general quality of care and patient satisfaction, and may be used retrospectively to evaluate the process or plan for future care. Outcomes do not directly assess process although they serve as an indicator that a process may be effective or ineffective, requiring further study or modification of process. Planners should focus on identifying three types of outcome measures:

- *Clinical*: Determines if there are positive results from clinical interventions.
- *Customer functioning*: Includes indicators of ability to perform.
- *Customer satisfaction*: Includes meeting expectations and needs.

Clinical/Critical Pathways

Clinical/critical pathway development is done by those involved in direct patient care. The pathway should require no additional staffing and cover the entire scope of an illness. Steps include:

- Selection of patient group and diagnosis, procedures, or conditions, based on analysis of data and observations of wide variance in approach to treatment and prioritizing organization and patient needs.
- Creation of interdisciplinary team of those involved in the process of care, including physicians, to develop pathway.
- Analysis of data includes literature review and study of best practices to identify opportunities for quality improvement.
- Identification of all categories of care, such as nutrition, medications, and nursing.
- Discussion, reaching consensus.
- Identifying the levels of care and number of days to be covered by the pathway.
- Pilot testing and redesigning steps as indicated.
- Educating staff about standards.
- Monitoring and tracking variances in order to improve pathways.

Clinical Problems and Research

Identifying clinical problems amenable to research is an evolving skill. Inexperienced nurses, especially those just starting out in nursing practice, are often looking to build information and skills because they lack experiential learning. They may research information about a disease or treatment that they are dealing with in order to have better skills and understanding. More experienced nurses, on the other hand, often look for information to improve patient outcomes, such as researching new procedures, treatments, or equipment for broader application. However, there is a need for both. Clinical inquiry is a program of questioning and evaluating practice through research and experience. It should include seeking a variety of data on a topic, evaluating the data, pooling results, and making determinations as to validity or applicability to the clinical practice. Clinical inquiry is also part of evidence-based practice in which data are used to support clinical decisions on an ongoing basis.

Critical Analysis

The nurse must be taught and understand the process of critical analysis and know how to conduct a survey of the literature. Basic concepts related to research include:

- *Survey of valid sources*: Information from a juried journal and an anonymous website or personal website are very different sources, and evaluating what constitutes a valid source of data is critical.
- *Evaluation of internal and external validity*: Internal validity shows a cause and effect relationship between two variables, with the cause occurring before the effect and no intervening variable. External validity occurs when results hold true in different environments and circumstances with different populations.
- *Sample selection and sample size*: Selection and size can have a huge impact on the results, but a sample that is too small may lack both internal and external validity. Selection may be so narrowly focused that the results cannot be generalized to others groups.

Critical Reading of Research Articles

There are a number of steps to critical reading to evaluate research:

- *Consider the source* of the material. If it is in the popular press, it may have little validity compared with something published in a juried journal.
- *Review the author's credentials* to determine if a person is an expert in the field of study.
- *Determine the thesis*, or the central claim of the research. It should be clearly stated.
- *Examine the organization* of the article, whether it is based on a particular theory, and the type of methodology used.
- *Review the evidence* to determine how it is used to support the main points. Look for statistical evidence and sample size to determine if the findings have wide applicability.
- *Evaluate* the overall article to determine if the information seems credible and useful and should be communicated to administration and/or staff.

Statistical Significance

Many research studies are most concerned with *internal validity*, adequate unbiased data properly collected and analyzed within the population studied, but studies that determine the efficacy of procedures or treatments, for example, should have *external validity* as well; that is, the results should be *generalizable* (true) for similar populations. *Replication* of the study with different subjects, researchers, and under different circumstances should produce similar results. For various reasons, some people may be excluded from a study so that instead of randomized subjects, the subjects may be highly selected. When data is compared with another population in which there is less or more selection, results may be different. The selection of subjects, in this case, would interfere with external validity. Part of the design of a study should include considerations of whether it should have external validity or whether there is value for the institution based solely on internal validation.

Selection bias occurs when the method of selecting subjects results in a cohort that is not representative of the target population because of inherent error in design. For example, if all infants who develop urinary infections are evaluated per urine culture and sensitivities for microbial resistance, but only those infants with clinically evident infections are included, a number of patients with subclinical infections may be missed, skewing the results. Selection bias is only a concern when participants in studies are specifically chosen. Many surveillance studies do not involve selection of subjects. *Information bias* occurs when there are errors in classification, so an estimate of association is incorrect. Nondifferential misclassification occurs when there is similar misclassification of disease or exposure among both those who are diseased/exposed and those who are not. Differential misclassification occurs when there is a differing misclassification of disease or exposure among both those who are diseased/exposed and those who are not.

Qualitative and Quantitative Data

Both qualitative and quantitative data are used for analysis, but the focus is quite different:

- Qualitative data: Data are described verbally or graphically, and the results are subjective, depending upon observers to provide information. Interviews may be used as a tool to gather information, and the researcher's interpretation of data is important. Gathering this type of data can be time-intensive, and it can usually not be generalized to a larger population. This type of information gathering is often useful at the beginning of the design process for data collection.
- Quantitative data: Data are described in terms of numbers within a statistical format. This type of information gathering is done after the design of data collection is outlined, usually in later stages. Tools may include surveys, questionnaires, or other methods of obtaining numerical data. The researcher's role is objective.

Hypothesis and Hypothesis Testing

A *hypothesis* should be generated about the probable cause of the disease/infection based on the information available in laboratory and medical records, epidemiologic study, literature review, and expert opinion. A hypothesis, for example, should include the infective agent, the likely source, and the mode of transmission: "Wound infections with *Staphylococcus aureus* were caused by reuse and inadequate sterilization of single-use irrigation syringes used during wound care in the ICU." *Hypothesis testing* includes data analysis, laboratory findings, and outcomes of environmental testing. It usually includes ***case*** control studies, with two to four controls picked for each case of infection. They may be matched according to age, sex, or other characteristics, but they are not infected at the time they are picked for the study. Cohort studies, whose controls are picked based on having or lacking exposure, may also be instituted. If the hypothesis cannot be supported, then a new hypothesis or different testing methods may be necessary.

Lifelong Learning

Lifelong learning requires commitment on the part of the nurse, the organization/facility, and the profession:

- *The nurse* must make an individual commitment to lifelong learning as a professional and ethical responsibility. This includes not only experiential learning but also formal learning, such as classes, and additional training.
- *The organization/facility* must give lifelong learning a priority focus, requiring that staff acquire ongoing education, both formal and informal. This commitment requires an allocation of resources to increase salaries, provide release time, and reimburse educational costs.
- *The profession* must continue to lobby legislatures throughout the United States to require that all licensed nurses complete continuing education courses to renew their licenses to practice. The profession, through professional organizations and the efforts of all nurses, must continue to set standards for certification and continue to delineate the evolving role of nurses as part of the health care team.

Evidence-Based Research

Evidence-based research is the use of current research and patient values in practice to establish a plan of care for each child. Research may be the result of large studies of best practices or individual research from observations in practice about the effectiveness of treatment. Evidence-based practice requires a commitment to ongoing research and outcomes evaluations. Many resources are available: Guide to Clinical Preventive Services by the Agency for Healthcare Research and Quality of the US Department of Health and Human Services (http://www.ahrq.gov/clinic/cps3dix.htm).

Evidence-based practice requires a thorough understanding of research methods in order to evaluate the results and determine if they can be generalized. Results must also be evaluated in terms of cost-effectiveness. Steps to evidence-based practice include:

- making a diagnosing
- researching and analyzing results
- applying research findings to plan of care
- evaluating outcomes

Incorporation of Research Findings

Incorporating research findings should be central to all work of the acute care nurse and should be routinely disseminated as part of practice, education, and consultation. Any time the nurse gives a presentation or provides written material, references should be made to research findings because this provides supporting evidence and lends credence to the information the nurse is providing. Often research can provide guidance for surveillance or interventions and give valuable insights. References that are used or referred to should always be properly cited so that the work of researchers is credited. If a presentation is given orally, then the nurse should prepare a list of references. Newsletters and e-mail or Internet reports and communications should include research highlights or summaries of current studies of interest, with links to online articles provided when possible to encourage people to read the research for themselves and become more knowledgeable about issues related to children.

Outcomes Evaluation

Outcomes evaluation is an important component of evidence-based practice, which involves both internal and external research. All treatments are subjected to review to determine if they produce positive outcomes, and policies and protocols for outcomes evaluation should be in place. Outcomes evaluation includes the following:

- *Monitoring* over the course of treatment involves careful observation and record keeping that notes progress, with supporting laboratory and radiographic evidence as indicated by condition and treatment.
- *Evaluating* results includes reviewing records as well as current research to determine if outcomes are within acceptable parameters.
- *Sustaining* involves continuing treatment, but continuing to monitor and evaluate.
- *Improving* means to continue the treatment but with additions or modifications in order to improve outcomes.
- *Replacing* the treatment with a different treatment must be done if outcomes evaluation indicates that current treatment is ineffective.

Performance Improvement Plan

The development of a performance improvement plan requires a number of steps, and while different approaches may be utilized, all should focus on quality planning, control, and improvement. Development may include:

- *Designing the process*: This includes creation of a team and establishing a process based on data, identifying customers, and assessing the ability of the organization to implement the plan. Training needs and resources should be included in the initial design.
- *Designing the plan*: This includes strategic planning for organization-wide participation and collaborative activities, which may be department/discipline specific or interdisciplinary. The plan must be consistent with vision and mission statements and goals and objectives. Performance expectations and measurements must be included.
- *Planning for implementation*: This includes defining quality, educating leadership and staff, writing the plan and including standards of care and guidelines, considering issues related to patient safety, and establishing benchmarks and outcomes measurements.

Assessment of Customer Needs

Surveys are valuable tools in assessing both progress and customer needs. However, care must be taken in the design of the survey if it is to have validity. A number of decisions must be made:

- *Target group*: Who will receive the survey? In some cases, an entire population of customers (all patients being discharged) may be targeted, but in other cases only a percentage will be done (30% of discharges from the emergency department). Identifying the target group can be complex.
- *Type of survey*: This may be paper, telephone, or Internet. There are different investments of time and money for each.
- *Type of questions*: Questions with a yes/no decision are usually easier to quantify than open-ended questions or scales, although scales are frequently used to assess degree of satisfaction.
- *Format*: This includes font size, color, general layout, and American Disability Act compliance.
- *Follow-up*: Reminders or incentives for people to complete surveys are needed, as completion rates are often low.

Epidemiological Issues

Incidence and prevalence surveillance are both hospital-wide surveillance methods. For example, *incidence* surveillance may include ongoing surveillance of infections of all hospitalized patients, recording the number of new infections in a population of patients over a specific period of time, so incidence surveillance is both time-consuming and expensive. However, it can identify clusters of infections and allows for risk-factor analysis.

The incidence rate:

(Numerator)	Number of new infections
(Denominator)	Total population in time period

Prevalence surveillance involves both *period prevalence*, which is a specific predetermined period of time for surveillance, and *point prevalence*, a specific point in time. Prevalence, then, is the number of case of nosocomial infections that are active during the period or point of time covered by the survey.

The prevalence rate:

(Numerator)	Number with active infection
(Denominator)	Total population in time period

Prevalence surveys are less time-consuming and expensive, but results can be skewed by random infections/events, resulting in overestimation.

Targeted Surveillance

Targeted surveillance is limited in scope, focusing on particular types of problems, areas in the facility, or patient population. It is less expensive than hospital-wide surveillance and may provide more meaningful data, but clusters of problems outside the survey parameters may be missed. Targeted areas are picked based on characteristics such as frequency of the disorder, mortality rates, financial costs, and the ability to use data to prevent the disorder:

- *Site-directed* targets particular sites of infection, such as bloodstream, wound, or urine.
- *Unit-directed* targets selected service areas of the hospital, such as intensive care units or neonatal units.
- *Population-directed* targets groups that are considered high-risk, such as transplantation patients and those undergoing other invasive procedures.
- *Limited periodic* combines hospital-wide surveillance of all infections for one month each quarter followed by site-directed targets for the rest of the quarter. This increases the chance of detecting clusters of infection, but those that fall outside of the hospital-wide surveillance months would still be missed.

CQI

Continuous Quality Improvement (CQI) emphasizes the organization and systems and processes within that organization rather than individuals. It recognizes internal customers (staff) and external customers (patients) and utilizes data to improve processes. CQI represents the concept that most processes can be improved. CQI uses the scientific method of experimentation to meet needs and improve services and utilizes various tools, such as brainstorming, multivoting, various charts and diagrams, storyboarding, and meetings. Core concepts include:

- Quality and success is meeting or exceeding internal and external customer's needs and expectations.
- Problems relate to processes, and variations in process lead to variations in results.
- Change can be in small steps.

Steps to CQI include:

- Forming a knowledgeable team.
- Identifying and defining measures used to determine success.
- Brainstorming strategies for change.
- Plan, collect, and utilize data as part of making decisions.
- Test changes and revise or refine as needed.

The Shewhart Cycle

The **Shewhart cycle (Plan-Do-Check-Act)** is a method of continuous improvement that is part of quality management and is used to evaluate care and solve problems:

- *Plan* involves identifying and analyzing a problem, clearly defining the problem, setting goals, and establishing a process that coordinates with coordinates with leadership. Extensive brainstorming, including fishbone diagrams, identifies problematic processes and lists current process steps. Data are collected and analyzed and root cause analysis is completed.
- *Do* involves generating solutions from which to select one or more and then implementing the solution on a trial basis.

- *Check* involves gathering and analyzing outcomes data to determine the effectiveness of the solution. If effective, then continue to *Act*; if not, return to *Plan* and pick a different solution.
- *Act* involves identifying changes that need to be done to fully implement solution, adopting solution, and continuing to monitor results while picking another improvement project.

Use of Is-Is Not

Is-Is Not is a method to identify root causes by determining what a problem/event is and what it is not. The purpose of Is-Is Not is to keep the team focused on the immediate problem. Steps include creating a table with the problem at the top and columns for "Is" and "Is Not" and filling in the table by doing the following:

- *Identifying what the problem/event IS:* Ask what, why, when, where, how, and how much in relation to the process rather than focusing on the people involved. Create a detailed description of the problem/event.
- *Identifying of what the problem/event IS NOT*: Ask what things could have caused the same problem but did not. Evaluate similar processes in which the problem did not occur.
- *Comparing*: The two columns of information are examined to determine what distinguishes them, helping to find potential causes
- *Identifying changes*: Note changes that may have occurred, resulting in the problem, leading to a root cause.

Root Cause Analysis

Root cause analysis (RCA) is a retrospective attempt to determine the cause of an event, often a sentinel event such as an unexpected death, or a cluster of events. RCA involves interviews, observations, and review of medical records. Often, an extensive questionnaire is completed by the person doing the RCA, tracing essentially every step in hospitalization and care, including every treatment, every medication, and every contact. The focus of the RCA is on systems and processes rather than individuals. How did the system break down? Where did the problem arise? In some cases, there may be one root cause, but in others, the causes may be multiple. The RCA also must include a thorough review of literature to ensure that action plans based on the results of the RCA reflect current best practices. Action plans without RCA may be nonproductive. If, for example, an infection were caused by contaminated air, action plans to increase disinfection of the operating room surfaces would not be effective.

Tracer Methodology

Tracer methodology is a method that looks at the continuum of care a patient receives from admission to postdischarge. A patient is selected to be "traced" and the medical record serves as a guide. Tracer methodology uses the experience of this patient to evaluate the processes in place through documents and interviews. For example, if a patient received physical therapy, surveyors may begin with the following:

- *Physical therapists*: How do they receive the orders and arrange patient transport? How is the therapy administered? How is progress noted?
- *Transport staff*: How do they receive requests? How long does transfer take? What routes do they use? How do they transport patients? How do they clean transport equipment? What do they do if emergency arises during transport?
- *Nursing staff*: How do they notify PT of orders? How do they prepare patients? How do they know the therapy schedule? How do they coordinate PT with the need for other treatments? How do they learn about patient progress?

Cost-Benefit Analysis

According to the CDC, a surgical site infection caused by *Staphylococcus aureus* results in an average of 12 additional days of hospitalization and costs $27,000. (In actuality, the cost may vary widely from one institution to another, so local data may be used.) A **cost-benefit analysis** uses average cost of problem (infection) and the cost of intervention to demonstrate savings. For example, if a surgical unit were averaging 10 surgical site infections annually, the cost would be:

10 x $27,000 = $270,000 annually.

If the interventions include new software ($10,000) for surveillance, an additional staff person ($65,000), benefits ($15,000), and increased staff education, including materials ($2,000), the total intervention cost would be:

$10,000 + $65,000 +$15,000 + $2,000 = $92,000

If the goal were to decrease infections by 50% to 5 infections per year, the savings would be calculated:

5 x $27,000 = $135,000

Subtracting the intervention cost from the savings:

$135,000 – $92,000 = $43,000 annual cost benefit.

Each year, about 2 million nosocomial infections result in 90,000 deaths and an estimated $6.7 billion in additional health costs. From that perspective, decreasing infections should reduce costs, but there are human savings in suffering as well, and it can be difficult to place a dollar value on that. A *cost-effective analysis* measures the effectiveness of an intervention rather than the monetary savings. If each infection adds about 12 days to hospitalization, then a reduction in infection by five would be calculated:

5 x 12 = 60 fewer patient-infection days.

Efficacy studies may compare a series of cost-benefit analyses to determine the intervention with the best cost-benefit. They may also be used for *process or product evaluation.* For example, a study might be done to determine the infection rates of four different types of catheters to determine which type resulted in the fewest infections, thus saving the most money (and infection days). *Incremental cost-effectiveness ratio* is the ratio of cost change to outcome change.

Recommendations for Practice Changes

Interventions and outcomes should be tied to each other. After an initial cost-benefit analysis and institution of an intervention, outcomes need to be assessed carefully to determine if the intervention is meeting the goal set for it and is cost-effective. If, for example, a hospital is investing $93,000 additionally each year to control infections, expecting a savings of five infections at $135,000 ($43,000 net), but in fact the savings amount to only two infections at $34,000, then the added cost to the hospital is $59,000. Changes in practice, however, cannot be made only on the basis of monetary figures. Further analysis must be done to determine if other variables affected the outcomes. If the hospital opened a transplant unit with additional surgical patients, then the reduction in two infections might be impressive. If there is a staph carrier among the staff, then this might account for additional infections. In some cases, a change of practice is required.

Communicating Research Results

There are a number of ways to communicate research results about procedures, products, or technology:

- Presentations to administration and those in positions of leadership, such as team leaders or managers, to garner support for incorporating findings into practice.
- Inservice training/education that focuses on results of research and explains applicability.
- Print distribution in the form of flyers or newsletters that outlines the research findings.
- Electronic newsletters or training modules that present the research findings.
- Discussions with intra- and interdisciplinary team members about the research and ways in which to apply those to the practice of care.

- Communicating is only one part of the process. Procedures must be in place in each organization that outline the steps to incorporating research findings into practice. An interdisciplinary team should evaluate the research findings and together create a system-wide approach to application, with the goal to improve outcomes for patients.

Response to Diversity

Response to Diversity

Response to diversity is the ability to recognize a wide range of differences (social, cultural, ethnic, racial, economic, language, religious), to appreciate these differences and incorporate consideration for them into the plan of care. Diverse groups also include the disabled persons, gay persons, and marginal groups, such as homeless persons. Levels of response to diversity include:

- Level 1: This nurse can assess diversity with standardized questionnaires and provide care based on a personal belief system and past experience, but does not seek assistance in dealing adequately with diversity.
- Level 3: This nurse takes a much more active role in asking about issues of diversity and incorporates needs into the plan of care, teaching the patient about the health care system.
- Level 5: This nurse considers issues of diversity in all aspects of care and presents patients with alternatives, responding to, anticipating, and integrating consideration of cultural and other differences.

Impact of Poverty

There are a number of issues that impact access to care, but poverty is one of the most significant and can affect care in many ways:

- Parents may not have health insurance and may not qualify for state medical assistance or may not be aware that they are eligible, so they do not take their children for routine medical visits.
- Practitioners may not accept state medical assistance payments because of low reimbursement rates, leaving parents with few options.
- Employers may not allow parents to take time off from work during the times that most practices are open to provide care, or the parents cannot afford to lose income, so most medical care is provided by emergency departments when a crisis arises.

Parents may lack automobiles or have insufficient funds for or access to public transportation to take a child to medical visits, especially in more rural areas.

Language Barriers

Language barriers often compromise patient's access to care and compliance with treatment, especially if the family is non-English speaking or has poor English skills. If the acute care nurse's practice draws from a minority population, then the nurse should consider proactive steps to resolving the issue of language barriers, such as hiring bilingual staff, taking language classes, or providing translated materials, such as treatment guidelines and pamphlets, or symbol-based signs. Many practices depend on family members, often children, to translate, but this is not a good solution as children often lack the maturity to assume this responsibility and may also lack the vocabulary or understanding to translate effectively, leading to serious misunderstandings. Interpreters should have training in medical vocabulary. In some cases, volunteer translators can be trained. Another solution is to pool translation resources among a number of practices so that costs are manageable.

Diversity Awareness

Issues of cultural diversity must be an integral part of the plan of care so that they are always addressed. Individuals vary considerably in their attitudes, so assuming that all members of an ethnic or cultural group share the same values is never valid. The individual must be assessed as well as the group. However, basic cultural guidelines should be available to staff, addressing issues such as eye contact, proximity, and gestures. It is important to take time to observe family dynamics and language barriers, arranging for translators if necessary to ensure that there is adequate communication. In patriarchal cultures, such as the Mexican culture, the eldest male may speak for the patient. In some Muslim cultures, females will resist care by males.

The attitudes and beliefs of the patient in relation to care and treatment must be understood, accepted, and treated with respect. In some cases, the use of healers or other cultural traditions must be incorporated into a plan of care.

Cultural Competence

Difference cultures view health and illness from very different perspectives, and patients often come from a mix of many cultures, so the acute care nurse must be not only accepting of cultural differences but must be sensitive and aware. There are a number of characteristics that are important for a nurse to have cultural competence:

- *Appreciating diversity*: This must be grounded in information about other cultures and understanding of their value system.
- *Assessing own cultural perspectives*: Self-awareness is essential to understanding potential biases.
- *Understanding intercultural dynamics*: This must include understanding ways in which cultures cooperate, differ, communicate, and reach understanding.
- *Recognizing institutional culture*: Each institutional unit (hospital, clinic, office) has an inherent set of values that may be unwritten but is accepted by the staff.
- *Adapting patient service to diversity*: This is the culmination of cultural competence as it is the point of contact between cultures.

Cultural Differences/Issues

Often health care providers who strive to be culturally competent are unaware that patients/families have very different perspectives about issues central to their health. According to the National Center for Cultural Competence there are a number of specific cultural differences/issues that health care providers should understand:

- Attitudes about illness and the cause of illness may be very different from one culture to another.
- Understanding of general health, mechanisms of healing, and issues of wellness may be very diverse.
- Attitudes about health care providers may range from very positive to very negative.
- The manner of help seeking for medical problems may vary, and health care providers may not recognize help-seeking behavior when it is not direct.
- Attitudes about traditional and nontraditional treatment influence the individual's medical choices.
- Attitudes of health care workers may project biases to which the patients are subjected.
- The current health system is often not culturally or linguistically diverse, so patient needs may be overlooked.

Tailoring Care to Diversity

Studies indicate that those who are diverse, that is ethnical, cultural, or lifestyle minorities, are often treated differently by health care providers in the sense that they may receive less than optimal care. It is incumbent on staff to ensure that all patients/families receive equal quality care but with delivery of care tailored to meet the individual needs of the patients. This begins with asking staff to assess their own attitudes and open discussion about differences to help people to gain self-awareness. This will help them determine if their ideas are stereotypical and/or based on lack of knowledge. The care plan should be formatted to specifically address diversity issues so that discussions of diversity and preferences are part of the care plan development and not an addendum. The original assessment should include questions about family, country of birth, educational level, religious preferences, and native language, with explanations as to why the questions are asked. This will establish a relationship of trust and respect that encourages the patient/family to express individual differences.

RESEARCH AND EXPERIENTIAL KNOWLEDGE

Acceptance and responsiveness to diversity requires an organizational commitment with ongoing inservice and training to assist staff. This may include:

- Multicultural advisory committees with community representatives to provide insight and determine areas for research or outreach to diverse groups.
- Mentors or consultants who can provide guidance to staff dealing with issues of diversity.
- Adaptation of patient/family materials for diverse groups, including patient information materials and surveys. These should be culturally appropriate and in various languages for those who are not proficient in English.
- Strategies to hire, retain, and promote a staff that is diverse and representative of the community.
- Training on how to work with interpreters.

Integrating cultural content throughout training curriculum, with specific information about cultural attitudes toward intimacy, sexuality, end-of-life, mental and physical illness, drug use, and health in general. Including a representative of diverse groups for presentations or group or panel discussions is particularly helpful.

PROFESSIONAL BOUNDARIES

Professional boundaries that show respect for the individual can be difficult to establish as part of delivery of care, especially with diverse populations because the nurse may unknowingly violate personal or spiritual values. Diverse groups include those on the fringes of society, such as homeless or abused persons. It is very important that nurses remain cognizant of the potential to abuse a position of power; the patient/family are in many ways dependent upon the nurse, and because of language, fears, or cultural constraints may not feel able to state their concerns. A relationship with a patient must be caring but at the same time professional and nonjudgmental. The needs of the patient/family must always be considered, and this may mean utilizing a translator to ensure that the patient/family are assuming an active role in the plan of care or making referrals to others in the health care or allied professions.

Belief Systems

JEHOVAH'S WITNESSES

Jehovah's Witnesses have traditionally shunned transfusions and blood products as part of their religious belief. In 2004, the *Watchtower,* a Jehovah Witness publication, presented a guide for members. When medical care indicates the need for blood transfusion or blood products and the patient and/or family members are practicing Jehovah's Witnesses, this may present a conflict. It is important to approach the patient/family with full information and reasons for the transfusion or blood components without being judgmental, allowing them to express their feelings. In fact, studies show that while adults often refuse transfusions for themselves, they frequently allow their children to receive blood products, so one should never assume that an individual would refuse blood products based on the religion alone. Jehovah's Witnesses can receive fractionated blood cells, thus allowing hemoglobin-based blood substitutes. The following guidelines are provided to church members:

Not acceptable	Whole blood: red cells, white cells, platelets, plasma
Acceptable	Fractions from red cells, white cells, platelets, and plasma

Facilitation of Learning

Teaching Implementation

The Synergy Model

Facilitation of learning is the ability to facilitate learning by patient and family/caregivers as well as other health and allied professionals and community members. Facilitation of learning requires needs assessment and preparation of content that is suited for the receiver in terms of delivery and content. Levels of facilitation of learning include:

- Level 1: This nurse is able to deliver planned educational content that is disease specific but does not have the ability to assess patient abilities or readiness to learn. The patient/family is considered a passive recipient of knowledge.
- Level 3: This nurse is able to individualize treatment according to patient/family needs and has an understanding of different methods of teaching and learning styles. The patient's needs are considered in planning.
- Level 5: This nurse has excellent understanding of teaching methods, learning styles, and assessment for learning readiness, and develops an educational plan in cooperation and collaboration with others, including patients, families, and other health care and allied professionals.

Assessing Educational Needs

There are a number of different methods that can be used to assess the educational needs of health care workers:

- Review job descriptions including the educational qualifications/certifications for all different levels of staff to determine what, realistically, they should be expected to know based on education.
- Review job orientation and training materials to determine what the staff has been taught.
- Conduct meetings with the staff in different departments to brainstorm areas of concern and potential training needs.
- Meet with team leaders and department heads for their input about the need for education.
- Administer short quizzes to staff asking about various topics of concern.
- Provide questionnaires to staff to obtain information about their own perceptions of what they know or need to know in terms of education.
- Make direct observations of staff.

Goals, Objectives, Lesson Plans

Once a topic for performance improvement education has been chosen, then goals, measurable objectives with strategies, and lesson plans must be developed. A class should stay focused on one area rather than trying to cover many things. For example:

Goal: increase compliance with hand hygiene standards in ICU.

Objectives:

- Develop series of posters and fliers by June 1.
- Observe 100% compliance with hand hygiene standards at 2 weeks, 1-month, and 2-month intervals after training is completed.

Strategies:

- Conduct 4 classes at different times over a 1-week period, May 25–31.
- Place posters in all nursing units, staff rooms, and utility rooms by January 3.
- Develop a slide show presentation for class and Intranet/Internet for access by all staff by May 25.
- Utilize handwashing kits.

Lesson plans:

- Discussion period: Why do we need 100% compliance?
- Slide Show: The case for hand hygiene.
- Discussion: What did you learn?
- Demonstration and activities to show effectiveness
- Handwashing technique.

Development, Implementation, and Evaluation

There are many approaches to teaching, and the nurse educator must prepare, present, and coordinate a wide range of educational workshops, lectures, discussions, and one-on-one instructions on any chosen topic. All types of classes will be needed, depending upon the purpose and material:

- *Educational workshops* are usually conducted with small groups, allowing for maximal participation, and are especially good for demonstrations and practice sessions.
- *Lectures* are often used for more academic or detailed information that may include questions and answers but limit discussion. An effective lecture should include some audiovisual support.
- *Discussions* are best with small groups so that people can actively participate. This is a good for problem solving.
- *One-on-one instruction* is especially helpful for targeted instruction in procedures for individuals.
- *Computer/Internet modules* are good for independent learners.

Participants should be asked to evaluate the presentations in the forms of surveys or suggestions, but ultimately the program is evaluated in terms of patient outcomes.

Audience Size

There are a number of issues related to audience size that must be considered when planning presentations.

- Class participation is more difficult in a large class because there may not be time for all to speak individually. Breaking the class into small groups or pairs for discussion for part of the class time can increase participation, but there must be a focused purpose to the discussion so that people stay on task.
- In small groups, placing chairs in a circle or sitting around a table allows people to look at each other and have more active discussions than if they are sitting in rows.

Online "virtual" classes can vary considerably in size, depending upon the type of presentation and whether or not scores and replies are automated or posted by the instructor. If a large group is taking an online course, setting up a "chat room" can facilitate exchange of ideas.

Handouts

Handouts are a fixture in classes, but many end up in the wastebasket without ever being used, so thought should be given to providing handouts that are useful:

- Handouts that simply copy a slide show presentation or repeat everything in the presentation are less helpful than those that summarize the main points.
- Giving out handouts immediately prior to a discussion ensures that most of the class will be looking at the handout instead of the speaker. Thus, handouts should be placed in a folder or binder and passed out before class so people can peruse them in advance, or passed out at the end of class.
- Handouts can be used to provide guidance or worksheets for small group discussions.
- Poster-type handouts (with drawings or pictures) that can be placed on bulletin boards are useful.
- Handouts should be easily readable and not smudged copies of newspaper articles or small print text.

Videos

Videos are a useful adjunct to teaching as they reduce the time needed for one-on-one instruction (increasing cost-effectiveness). Passive presentation of videos, such as in the waiting area, has little value, but focused viewing in which the nurse discusses the purpose of the video presentation prior to viewing and then is available for discussion after viewing can be very effective. Patients and/or families are often nervous about understanding patient care and are unsure of their abilities, so they may not focus completely when the nurse is presenting information. Allowing the patients/families to watch a video demonstration or explanation first and allowing them to stop or review the video presentation can help them to grasp the fundamentals before they have to apply them, relieving some of the anxiety they may be experiencing. Videos are much more effective than written materials for those with low literacy or poor English skills. The nurse should always be available to answer questions and discuss the material after the patients/families finish viewing.

Readability

Studies have indicated that learning is more effective if oral presentations and/or demonstrations are supplemented with reading materials, such as handouts. Readability (the grade level of material) is a concern because many patients and families may have limited English skills or low literacy, and it can be difficult for the nurse to assess a person's reading level. The average American reads effectively at the 6th to 8th grade level (regardless of education achieved), but many health education materials have a much higher readability level. Additionally, research indicates that even people with much higher reading skills learn medical and health information most effectively when the material is presented at the 6th to 8th grade readability level. Therefore, patient education materials (and consent forms) should not be written at higher than 6th to 8th grade level. Readability index calculators are available on the Internet to give an approximation of grade level and difficulty. These can be used to prepare materials without expertise in teaching reading.

Advising and Relaying Changes

Changes in policies, procedures, or working standards are common and the quality professional is responsible for educating the staff about changes related to processes, which should be communicated to staff in an effective and timely manner:

- *Policies* are usually changed after a period of discussion and reviewed by administration and staff, so all staff should be made aware of policies under discussion. Preliminary information regarding the issue should be disseminated to staff during meetings or through printed notices.
- *Procedures* may be changed to increase efficiency or improve patient safety often as the result of surveillance and data about outcomes. Procedures changes are best communicated in workshops with demonstrations. Posters and handouts should be available as well.
- *Working standards* are often changed because of regulatory or accrediting requirements and this information should be covered extensively in a variety of different ways, such as discussions, workshops, or handouts, so that the implications are clearly understood.

Physical Environment

A number of issues must be considered when teaching a course and determining the appropriate audiovisuals and handout materials. **The physical environment** is a major consideration, especially when using audiovisual material.

- First, everyone in the room must be able to hear and see. In a small room, a television screen may suffice, but in a large space, a projection screen must be used.
- Another issue is lighting. Some projectors have low resolution and the lights need to be dimmed or turned off or windows covered. Turning lights on and off a dozen times during a presentation can be very distracting. A small portable light at a speaker podium or an alternate presentation can be used.
- Text size for presentations is another issue: slide shows or other presentations that include text must be of sufficient font size to be read from the back of the room.

Visual-Auditory-Kinesthetic Model

Not all people are aware of their preferred **learning style**. A range of teaching materials/methods that relates to all 3 learning preferences, visual, auditory, and kinesthetic, should be available and appropriate for different ages. Part of assessment for teaching involves choosing the right approach based on observation and feedback. Often, presenting learners with different options gives a clue to their preferred learning style. Some people have a combined learning style:

Visual learners learn best by seeing and reading:

- Provide written directions or picture guides, or demonstrate procedures.
- Use charts and diagrams.
- Provide photos or videos.

Auditory learners learn best by listening and talking:

- Procedures while demonstrating and have learner repeat.
- Plan extra time to discuss and answer questions.
- Provide audiotapes.

Kinesthetic learners learn best by handling, doing, and practicing.

- Provide hands-on experience throughout teaching.
- Encourage handling of supplies/equipment.
- Allow learner to demonstrate.
- Minimize instructions and allow person to explore equipment and procedures.

Learning Styles

Recognizing and applying teaching methods to learning styles can improve learning markedly, but the instructor should keep a number of principles of dealing with learning styles in mind:

- Learning styles can and should be assessed for both the instructor and the patient family. People often can state a preference when asked how they best learn. If the nurse understands his/her own learning style, it can help the nurse understand its importance in teaching and learning.
- The nurse must use care to not prepare most educational materials to match his/her own learning style but to remember that other types of material must also be prepared.
- Helping the patient/family to understand their learning styles can make them more efficient learners.
- Materials that address more than one learning style (audio plus visual, for example) can help learners adapt learning to various types of presentations.

Educational materials can be adapted to appeal to different learning styles.

Principles of Adult Learning

Adults have a wealth of life and/or employment experiences. Their attitudes toward education may vary considerably. There are, however, some principles of adult learning and typical characteristics of adult learners that an instructor should consider when planning strategies for teaching parents, families, or staff:

- *Practical and goal-oriented:*
  - Provide overviews or summaries and examples.
  - Use collaborative discussions with problem-solving exercises.
  - Remain organized with the goal in mind.
- *Self-directed:*
  - Provide active involvement, asking for input.
  - Allow different options toward achieving the goal.
  - Give them responsibilities.
- *Knowledgeable:*
  - Show respect for their life experiences/education.
  - Validate their knowledge and ask for feedback.
  - New material to information with which they are familiar.
- *Relevancy-oriented:*
  - How information will be applied.
  - Clearly identify objectives.
- *Motivated:*
  - Provide certificates of professional advancement and/or continuing education credit for staff when possible.

Review Video: Adult Learning Processes and Theories
Visit mometrix.com/academy and enter code: 638453

Models and Theories

The Health Belief Model

The Health Belief Model (HBM) is a model used to predict health behavior with the understanding that people take a health action to avoid negative consequences if the person expects that the negative outcome can be avoided and that he/she is able to do the action. The HBM, as modified, is based on six basic perceptions:

- Susceptibility: Belief that the person may get a negative condition.
- Severity: Understanding of how serious a condition is.
- Benefit: Belief that the action will reduce risk of getting the condition.
- Barriers: Direct and psychological costs involved in taking action.
- Action cues: Strategies used to encourage action, such as education.
- Self-efficacy: Confidence in the ability to take action and achieve positive results.

This model attempts to encourage people to make changes or take action (such as stopping smoking) in order to avoid negative consequences, so this model, when used for education, focuses on the negative consequences (such as quitting smoking to avoid cardiovascular and pulmonary disease).

Review Video: What is the Health Belief Model?
Visit mometrix.com/academy and enter code: 954833

Theory of Reasoned Action

The Theory of Reasoned Action, developed in 1975 by Martin Fishbein and Icek Ajzen, is based on the idea that the actions people take voluntarily can be predicted according to their personal attitude toward the action and their perception of how others will view their doing the action. There are three basic concepts to the theory:

- *Attitudes*: These are all of the attitudes about an action, and they may be weighted (some more important than others).
- *Subjective norms*: People are influenced by those in their social realm (family, friends) and their attitudes toward particular actions. The influence may be weighted. For example, the attitude of a spouse may carry more weight than the attitude of a neighbor.
- *Behavioral intention*: The intention to take action is based on weighing attitudes and subjective norms (opinions of others), resulting in a choice to either take an action or avoid the action.

Theory of Planned Behavior

The Theory of Planned Behavior, by Ajzen, evolved from the Theory of Reasoned Action in 1985 when studies showed that behavioral intention does not necessarily result in action. The Theory of Planned Behavior is more successful in predicting behavior. To the basic concepts of attitudes, subjective norms, and behavioral intentions encompassed by the earlier theory, Ajzen added the concept of *perceived behavioral control*, which relates to the individual's attitudes about self-efficacy and outcomes. Ajzen's theory shows that beliefs are central:

- Behavioral beliefs lead to attitudes toward a behavior/action.
- Normative beliefs lead to subjective norms.
- Control beliefs lead to perceived behavioral control.

All of these beliefs interact to influence intention and action. Basically, this theory relates to the person's confidence, based on beliefs and social influence of others, that he/she can actually do an action and that the outcome of this action will be positive. This theory looks at the power of emotions such as apprehension or fear when predicting behavior.

Stress Appraisal and Coping Theory

The transactional Stress Appraisal and Coping Theory is used to evaluate how people cope with stressors by going through a series of appraisals, based on personal ideas and resources (social, cultural) available to the person:

- *Primary appraisal*: The person considers and evaluates the importance of a current or future event that has resulted in stress.
- *Secondary appraisal*: The person considers his/her ability to control the stressor and to cope with it in terms of personal and social resources.
- *Coping*: The person develops strategies based on the primary and secondary appraisal in order to attempt to change the stressor or to think about the stressor in a different way.
- *Meaningful coping*: The person uses coping processes that lead to positive emotions in order to continue coping.
- *Outcomes*: The person sees the results of coping.
- *Disposition:* Some people tend to have positive expectations, others look for information, and still others seek avoidance, and these differences in disposition affect coping.

Family Systems Theory

Dr. Murray Bowen's Family Systems Theory suggests that one must look at the person in terms of his/her family unit because the members of a family have different roles and behavioral patterns, so a change in one person's behavior will affect the others in the family. There are eight interrelated concepts:

- *Triangle theory*: Two people comprise a basic unit, but when conflict occurs, a third person is drawn into the unit for stability with the resulting dynamic of two supporting one or two opposing one. This, in turn, draws in other triangles.
- *Self-differentiation*: People vary in need for external approval.
- *Nuclear family patterns*: Marital conflict, one spouse dysfunctional, one or more children impaired, and emotional distance.
- *Projection within a family*: Problems (emotional) passed from parent to child.
- *Transmission (multigenerational)*: Small differences in transmission from parent to child.
- *Emotional isolation*: Reducing or eliminating family contact.
- *Sibling order*: Influence on behavior and development.
- *Emotional process (society)*: Results in regressive or progressive social movements.

Transtheoretical Model

The Transtheoretical Model focuses on changes in behavior based on the individual's (not society's or others') decisions and is used to develop strategies to promote changes in health behavior. This model outlines stages people go through changing problem behavior and having a positive attitude about change. Stages of change:

- *Precontemplation*: The person is either unaware or under-informed about consequences of a problem behavior and has no intention of changing behavior in the next 6 months.
- *Contemplation*: The person is aware of costs and benefits of changing behavior and intends to change in the next 6 months but is procrastinating and not ready for action.
- *Preparation*: The person has a plan and intends to instigate change in the near future (1 month or less) and is ready for action plans.
- *Action*: The person is modifying behavior. Behavior change occurs only if behavior meets a set criterion (such as complete abstinence from drinking).
- *Maintenance*: The person works to maintain changes and gains confidence that he/she will not relapse.

Theory Application

The Transtheoretical Model stages of change (precontemplation, contemplation, preparation, action, and maintenance) are a process that the individual goes through in order to change behavior and attitudes, but there are other aspects to be considered. There are two temporal dimensions to this process:

- *Distance* of the behavior (from the time the process begins to the time change is made) is an important consideration.
- *Duration* of behavior (the time from change to relapse) is also important. Duration should become longer with a goal of no relapse.

Additionally, the model recognizes that there are *intervening variables*: decisional balance (the costs and benefits of change), self-efficacy (confidence in being able to change), and any other variables, such as social, environmental, psychological, or medical, that may affect behavior and change.

During each stage of the process of the Transtheoretical Model, people go through 10 processes of change as they attempt to modify their behavior:

- *Consciousness raising*: Seeking information
- *Counterconditioning*: Substituting alternative action for problem behavior, such as using relaxation techniques, positive statements, and desensitization.

- *Dramatic relief*: Expressing feelings (positive and negative) about change of problem behavior and solutions.
- *Environmental reevaluation*: Determining the effect the problem behavior has on others and developing empathy.
- *Helping relationships*: Accepting assistance from other to effectuate change.
- *Reinforcement management*: Accepting reward (from self or others) for changing problem behavior.
- *Self-liberation*: Believing change is possible and committing to change.
- *Self-reevaluation*: Reevaluating values in relation to problem behavior.
- *Social liberation*: Becoming aware (emotionally and cognitively) of positive lifestyles and feeling empowered.
- *Stimulus control*: Controlling situations in which problem behavior is triggered.

Bloom's Taxonomy

Bloom's taxonomy outlines behaviors that are necessary for learning, and this can apply to health care. The theory describes three types of learning:

- Cognitive (Learning and gaining intellectual skills to master 6 categories of effective learning.) Knowledge, Comprehension, Application, Analysis, Synthesis, Evaluation
- Affective (Recognizing 5 categories of feelings and values from simple to complex. This is slower to achieve than cognitive learning.)
    - Receiving phenomena: Accepting need to learn.
    - Responding to phenomena: Taking active part in care.
    - Valuing: Understanding value of becoming independent in care.
    - Organizing values: Understanding how surgery/treatment has improved life. Internalizing values: Accepting condition as part of life, being consistent and self-reliant.
- Psychomotor (Mastering 6 motor skills necessary for independence. This follows a progression from simple to complex.)
    - Perception: Uses sensory information to learn tasks.
    - Set: Shows willingness to perform tasks.
    - Guided response: Follows directions.
    - Mechanism: Does specific tasks.
    - Complex overt response: Displays competence in self-care.
    - Adaptation: Modifies procedures as needed.
    - Origination: Creatively deals with problems.

Effectiveness Evaluation

Education, like all interventions, must be evaluated for effectiveness. Two determinants of effectiveness include:

- *Behavior modification* involves thorough observation and measurement, identifying behavior that needs to be changed and then planning and instituting interventions to modify that behavior. An ACNP can use a variety of techniques, including demonstrations of appropriate behavior, reinforcement, and monitoring, until new behavior is adopted consistently. This is especially important when longstanding procedures and habits of behavior are changed.
- *Compliance rates* are often determined by observation, which should be done at intervals and on multiple occasions, but with patients, this may depend on self-reports. Outcome is another measure of compliance; that is, if education is intended to improve patient health and reduce risk factors and those occur, it is a good indication that there is compliance. Compliance rates are calculated by determining the number of events/procedures and degree of compliance.

Learner Outcomes

When the quality professional plans an educational offering, whether it be a class, an online module, a workshop, or educational materials, the professional should identify learner outcomes, which should be conveyed to the learners from the very beginning so that they are aware of the expectations. The subject matter of the educational material and the learner outcomes should be directly related. For example, if the quality professional is giving a class on decontamination of the environment, then a learner outcome might be: "Identify the difference between disinfectants and antiseptics." There may be one or multiple learner outcomes, but part of the assessment at the end of the learning experience should be to determine if, in fact, the learner outcomes have been achieved. A survey of whether or not the learners felt that they had achieved the learner outcomes can give valuable feedback and guidance to the quality professional.

Learning in Clinical Setting

The AACN Synergy Model

Septic shock is most common in newborns, those older than 50 years of age, and those who are immunocompromised. There is no specific test to confirm a diagnosis of septic shock, so diagnosis is based on clinical findings and tests that evaluate hematologic, infectious, and metabolic states: CBC, DIC panel, electrolytes, liver function tests, BUN, creatinine, blood glucose, ABGs, urinalysis, ECG, radiographs, and blood and urine cultures.

Treatment must be aggressive and includes:

- oxygen and endotracheal intubation as necessary
- IV access with 2-large bore catheters and central venous line
- rapid fluid administration at 0.5 L NS or isotonic crystalloid every 5 to 10 minutes as needed (to 4 to 6 L) (children: 10 mL/kg to total 60 mL/kg)
- monitoring urinary output to optimal greater than 30 mL/h (1 mL/h for children)
- inotropes (dopamine, dobutamine, norepinephrine) if no response to fluids or fluid overload
- empiric IV antibiotic therapy (usually with 2 broad spectrum antibiotics for both gram-positive and gram-negative bacteria) until cultures return and antibiotics may be changed
- hemodynamic and laboratory monitoring
- removing source of infection (abscess, catheter).

Levels of Outcomes

The AACN synergy model is based on three levels of quality outcomes (patient, nurse, and system). Six general *indicators of quality outcomes* include:

- satisfaction of patient and family
- adverse incidents rates
- rate of complications
- adherence to discharge plans
- mortality rate
- length of stay in hospital.

These general outcomes are based on outcomes derived from the patient, the nurse, and the system:

- *Patient outcomes* include functional change, behavioral change, trust, ratings, satisfaction, comfort, and quality of life.
- *Nurse outcomes* include physiological changes, presence or absence of complications, and extent to which care of treatment objectives were attained.
- *System outcomes* include recidivism, costs, and resource utilization.

Resiliency

Resiliency is the ability of the patient to utilize coping mechanisms and to recover. There are many factors that affect a patient's resiliency, ranging from personality and drive to family resources and support systems. Adults who are resilient tend to be more physically active and have the ability to find meaning in life, regardless of their circumstances. People who are depressed tend to have less resiliency. In children, high self-esteem and good temperaments correlate with resiliency while poverty and parental absence correlates with poor resiliency. Levels of resiliency include:

- Level 1: This patient has few reserves and is not able to adequately utilize coping mechanisms to deal with illness or recovery.
- Level 3: This patient has a moderate ability to cope and can deal effectively with some aspects of illness and recovery.
- Level 5: This patient has excellent coping mechanisms, as well as the ability to endure illness, and the drive to recover.

Vulnerability

Vulnerability is the patient's susceptibility to negative forces, such as stress or threats, that can affect outcomes. There are many factors that relate to vulnerability, and they may be quite individualized, but dependency, lack of adequate information about health status and care procedures, and poor relationship with care providers tend to increase vulnerability. Levels of vulnerability include:

- Level 1: This patient is very vulnerable and has little sense of protection or control and remains essentially dependent and fragile.
- Level 3: This patient is moderately vulnerable and has some sense of protection and control but remains dependent and fragile to some extent.
- Level 5: This patient has little vulnerability and has a strong sense of personal protection and control and is able to think and act independently toward achieving positive health outcomes.

Stability

Stability is the ability to maintain a steady-state equilibrium in the face of health challenges. Stability often relates to traditional medical characteristics (such as hemodynamic status) and measurements (such as blood pressure), those things that usually directly affect morbidity and mortality. Stability correlates with response to therapy. Stability relates to other patient characteristics, such as vulnerability and resiliency. Levels of stability include:

- Level I: This patient has a high risk of increased morbidity and mortality because of labile condition and poor response to therapy.
- Level 3. This patient is moderately stable for limited periods of time, and there is some response to therapy so risk for increased morbidity and mortality is reduced but not eliminated.
- Level 5: This patient is very stable, responds well to therapy, and has little risk for increased morbidity or mortality.

Complexity

Complexity occurs when two or more systems are entangled and complicating the patient's care and progress. Complexity can be viewed from a number of different perspectives: medical complexity in which more than one disease process is occurring, treatment complexity in which multiple treatments are required, or psychosocial complexity in which family roles/responsibilities are challenged. Levels of complexity include:

- Level 1: This patient faces an extremely complex situation and may have to deal with complicated family dynamics and/or a confusing medical presentation that cannot be easily quantified or managed.

- Level 3: This patient faces a moderately complex situation. Family dynamics may be somewhat unstable and clinical presentation may have some ambiguity.
- Level 5: This patient faces minimal complexity in family dynamic and/or clinical presentation.

Resource Availability

Resource availability is the extent of resources available to the patient. These resources may encompass a wide variety, including personal (religious or other beliefs, personality, strength of character, tolerance for pain), financial (personal or family income and fiscal resources), social (friends, coworkers, community, social status, social stability), psychological (emotional stability), and technical (knowledge and skills). With infants, children, and disabled or elderly patients, the resources available may be those of the parents, children, or other family members or caregivers, rather than the individual.

Levels of resource availability include:

- Level 1: This patient lacks adequate resources, often in many areas, including financial and personal, and may have inadequate knowledge to deal with illness effectively.
- Level 3: This patient has moderate resources but limitations remain, and resources may be weaker in some areas than in others.
- Level 5: This patient has excellent resources with strengths across multiple areas, such as adequate financial resources, good support systems, and excellent knowledge and skills

Participation in Care

Participation in care is the extent to which the family, patient, or caregivers are able or willing to participate in patient care. Participation in care encompasses a range of physical and clinical care, such as changing dressings; assisting with physical therapy; administering medications, such as pain control; and providing treatments, such as dialysis. Patients and parents/caregiver may vary in the degree of participation that they want, and this can be influenced by many factors, including education, knowledge, time pressures, and the attitudes of nurses and other staff. Patients and family may want to choose their level of participation. Levels of participation in care include:

- Level 1: This patient and/or family/caregivers do not participate in care at all because they are unable to do so or prefer not to.
- Level 2: This patient and/or family/caregivers participate in care to a moderate degree but are not independent and require ongoing assistance.
- Level 3: This patient and/or family/caregivers participate fully in care.

Participation in Decision Making

Participation in decision making is the extent to which the patient and/or family/caregivers participate in decisions about different aspects of treatment and care. The degree to which people want to make decisions can vary according to willingness, age, ethnicity, and social situation. There are often many options for care, and patients/families should be prepared with adequate information and support from health care providers in order to relieve the anxiety involved in making decisions. Children should be allowed input into decisions whenever possible, depending upon the age and maturity of the child. Levels of participation in decision making include:

- Level 1: This patient/family has no participation in decision making and is unable to participate, requiring others make decisions.
- Level 3: This patient/family has a moderate ability to make decisions with advice and guidance from health care providers or others, such as friends or other family.
- Level 5: This patient/family is able to make informed decisions.

Predictability

Predictability is the sum of characteristics that allows one to expect a patient to follow a certain course based on these characteristics. Predictability is used to determine outcomes and the likelihood of complications as well as staffing parameters. Numerous prediction models have been developed for various health conditions. Predictability may relate treatment outcomes or discharge outcomes. Evidence-based clinical pathways rely on predictability for different patient populations to determine the best methods to achieve an expected outcome. Different levels of predictability include:

- Level 1: This patient's course is not predictable because the illness or patient does not fit the usual parameters or because of unexpected events or outcomes.
- Level 3: This patient's course is moderately predictable with some occasional unexpected events or outcomes.
- Level 5: This patient's course is very predictable and follows that common to others in the same population.

Clinical Judgment

Clinical judgment is using clinical reasoning, decision making, and critical thinking to evaluate a situation and apply skills related to education, experience, knowledge, and evidence-based guidelines in providing care. Clinical judgment includes a thorough knowledge of the nursing process and ability to utilize data and research. Clinical judgment includes the use of intuition, based on experience, and a holistic understanding of all issues involved. Levels of clinical judgment include:

- Level 1: This nurse is at a beginner level and follows algorithms and pathways but cannot vary care according to needs, is able to collect only basic data, and defers to others for some decision making.
- Level 3: This nurse is competent in collecting and assessing data and can anticipate needs and manage patient care but recognizes when to ask for guidance.
- Level 5: This nurse is expert and able to process multiple sources of data and make reasoned decisions about patient care based on knowledge and experience and a holistic view of the patient's needs.

Advocacy/Moral Agency

Nurse competencies include advocacy/moral agency:

- *Advocacy* is working for the best interests of the patient despite personal values in conflict, and assisting patients so they have access to appropriate resources.
- *Agency* is openness and recognition of issues and a willingness to act.
- *Moral agency* is the ability to recognize needs and take action to influence the outcome of a conflict or decision.

The levels of advocacy/moral agency include:

- Level 1: This nurse works on behalf of the patient, assesses personal values, has awareness of patient's rights and ethical conflicts, and advocates for the patient when consistent with the nurse's personal values.
- Level 3: This nurse advocates for the patient/family, incorporates their values into the care plan even when they differ from the nurse's, and can utilize internal resources to assist patient/family with complex decisions.
- Level 3: This nurse advocates for patient/family despite differences in values and is able to utilize both internal and external resources to help to empower patient/family to make decisions.

Formal and Informal

Both formal and informal intra- and interdisciplinary education is necessary to improve patient outcomes and quality of care:

- *Formal education* comprises classes, workshops, and scheduled training. Participants are generally advised in advance and come prepared to learn about a particular topic. Formal education is often the best way to communicate complex information that needs media support, such as slide show presentations. Formal education is also cost-effective because many people can be served at one time.
- *Informal education* is equally valuable and can occur at any time. Many opportunities occur in the course of a day to provide informal education through mentoring, role modeling, discussing, and answering questions. Instituting dialogue with other nurses by asking for opinions or commenting on issues related to patient care often provides an opportunity to share information in a nonthreatening environment.

One-on-One Versus Group

Both one-on-one instruction and group instruction have a place in patient/family education.

- *One-on-one instruction* is the most costly for an institution because it is time intensive. However, it allows the patient and family more interaction with the nurse instructor, and allows the patient/family to have more control over the process by asking questions or having the instructor repeat explanations or demonstrations. One-on-one instruction is especially valuable when patients and families must learn particular skills, such as managing dialysis, or if confidentiality is important.
- *Group instruction* is the less costly because the needs of a number of people can be met at one time. Group presentations are more planned and usually scheduled for a particular time period (an hour, for example), so patients and families have less control. Questioning is usually more limited and may be done only at the end. Group instruction allows patients/families with similar health problems to interact. Group instruction is especially useful for general types of instruction, such as managing diet or other lifestyle issues.

Learning Readiness

The patient/family's readiness to learn should be assessed because if they are not ready, instruction is of little value. Often readiness is indicated when the patient/family asks questions or shows an interest in procedures. A number of factors are related to readiness to learn:

- *Physical factors*: A number of physical factors can affect ability. Manual dexterity may be required to complete a task, and this varies by age and condition. Hearing or vision deficits may impact ability. Complex tasks may be too difficult for some because of weakness or cognitive impairment, and modifications of the environment may be needed. Health status, age, and gender may all impact the ability to learn.
- *Experience*: A person's experience with learning can vary widely and is affected by his or her ability to cope with changes, personal goals, motivation to learn, and cultural background. People may have widely divergent ideas about what constitutes illness and/or treatment. Lack of English skills may make learning difficult and prevent people from asking questions.
- *Mental/Emotional status*: The support system and motivation may impact readiness. Anxiety, fear, or depression about the condition can make learning very difficult because the patient/family cannot focus on learning. The nurse must spend time to reassure the patient/family and wait until they are emotionally more receptive.
- *Knowledge/Education*: The knowledge base of the patient/family, their cognitive ability, and their learning styles all affect their readiness to learn. The nurse should always begin by assessing what knowledge the patient/family already has about their disease, condition, or treatment, and then build from that base. People with little medical experience may lack knowledge of basic medical terminology, which will interfere with their ability and readiness to learn.

ACNPC Practice Test

Want to take this practice test in an online interactive format?
Check out the online resources page, which includes interactive practice questions and much more: **mometrix.com/resources719/acnpc**

1. Parenteral nutrition with a total nutrient admixture that includes lipids has been ordered for a burn patient for administration over a 24-hour period. When preparing to administer the solution, the nurse practitioner observes that the oil has separated, forming an obvious layer. The nurse practitioner should take which of the following actions?

a. Administer the solution, as oil separation is normal.
b. Mix the solution by shaking the bag until no oil separation is noticeable.
c. Discard the solution.
d. Return the solution to the pharmacy for the addition of an emulsifier.

2. A 30-year-old patient complains of postoperative pain of 8 on a 1–10 scale 12 hours after surgery, although the patient is not moaning, grimacing, or exhibiting signs of pain. The patient last received pain medication 6 hours earlier and has orders for morphine every 4 hours as needed and ibuprofen every 6 hours as needed. Which of the following actions is most appropriate?

a. Give ibuprofen.
b. Give morphine.
c. Give ibuprofen, and if there is no relief in 1 hour, give morphine.
d. Question family members about the patient's pain tolerance before making a decision.

3. A 70-year-old patient with a fracture of the proximal femur develops sudden onset of hypoxia, tachypnea, high fever, buccal and conjunctival petechiae, and tachycardia 24 hours after injury. Initial arterial blood gases indicate respiratory alkalosis. Which of the following possible complications is the most likely cause of these symptoms?

a. Venous thromboembolism
b. Infection
c. Hemorrhage
d. Fat embolism syndrome

4. A 19-year-old male patient identifies himself as a homosexual and states that he wants his partner to visit him in the hospital; however, the patient's parents, who are paying the medical bills, state that the patient's partner may not visit. The nurse practitioner should do which of the following?

a. Allow the patient's partner to visit.
b. Tell the patient's partner he may not visit.
c. Ask the parents to reconsider.
d. Refer the issue to the ethics committee.

5. A patient with cirrhosis and portal hypertension is awaiting a liver transplant but has refractory ascites. The treatment of choice is

a. a peritoneovenous shunt.
b. a transjugular intrahepatic shunt.
c. diuretics.
d. paracentesis.

6. In a research project, some patients are excluded from the project; thus, the subjects are highly selected not randomized. This type of selection may result in results that primarily have

a. generalizability.
b. replicability.
c. external validity.
d. internal validity.

7. A patient with systemic lupus erythematosus has developed swollen, tender joints; increased fatigue and weakness; low-grade fever; mild depression; and loss of appetite. She has a rash on her face. Laboratory findings indicate an increased erythrocyte sedimentation rate. The most likely initial treatment is

a. immunosuppressive agents.
b. steroids only.
c. nonsteroidal anti-inflammatory drugs and corticosteroids.
d. antidepressants.

8. A patient with acute lung injury has crackling rales, tachypnea, and cyanosis. Oxygen therapy is instituted to maintain oxygen saturation at

a. $\geq 85\%$.
b. $> 90\%$.
c. $> 95\%$.
d. $\geq 98\%$.

9. Which of the following is a barrier to systems thinking?

a. Reliance on past experience
b. Identification with purpose
c. Strong consensus
d. Adaptability

10. A postoperative patient develops disseminated intravascular coagulation with bleeding from operative and puncture sites, gastrointestinal bleeding with distention and bloody diarrhea, petechiae, purpura, hypotension, and acute symptoms of shock. Expected laboratory findings include which of the following?

a. Decreased prothrombin and partial prothrombin times and increased platelet count and fibrinogen
b. Prolonged prothrombin and partial prothrombin times, increased platelet count, and decreased fibrinogen
c. Prolonged prothrombin and partial prothrombin times and decreased platelet count and fibrinogen
d. Decreased prothrombin and partial prothrombin times and decreased platelet count and increased fibrinogen

11. A patient is admitted to the unit after vomiting excessively for 4 days at home. The patient's serum pH is elevated; the partial pressure of carbon dioxide is relatively normal; and the urine pH is over 6. The patient is dizzy, confused, and exhibiting tremors, seizures, tingling, tachycardia, arrhythmias, and hypoventilation. The patient is most likely exhibiting symptoms of

a. respiratory alkalosis.
b. metabolic alkalosis.
c. respiratory acidosis.
d. metabolic acidosis.

12. In response to a recent increase in surgical site mortality rates in a hospital unit, which of the following methods is indicated to determine the cause?

a. External benchmarking
b. Targeted surveillance
c. Plan-Do-Check-Act
d. Root-cause analysis

13. A 40-year-old woman with type 1 diabetes presents with hyperventilation, dehydration with diuresis, increased thirst, and cardiac arrhythmias. Initial treatment is most likely to include

a. diazoxide to inhibit the release of insulin.
b. fluid (glucose) for hypoglycemia and electrolyte therapy for dehydration.
c. insulin therapy for ketoacidosis, fluid (nonglucose) therapy, and electrolyte replacement.
d. intravenous glucose solution for hypoglycemia.

14. A 62-year-old man with pancreatitis received narcotic medications to reduce pain. He experienced nausea and vomiting, and his abdomen became distended and uncomfortable. He has an absence of flatulence and bowel sounds. The most likely diagnosis is

a. bowel obstruction.
b. paralytic ileus.
c. bowel infarction.
d. short gut syndrome.

15. A patient who is being treated for renal failure exhibits ventricular arrhythmia with increasing electrocardiographic changes, weakness with ascending paralysis, hyperreflexia, diarrhea, and increased confusion. The patient most likely has

a. hyperkalemia.
b. hypokalemia.
c. hypocalcemia.
d. hypercalcemia.

16. A 40-year-old patient who suffered a traumatic brain injury is in a vegetative state and is maintained on life support. The patient's husband has a health care power of attorney for the patient, but he is estranged and living separately. A decision regarding continuation of life support must be made, but the family members cannot agree. Who has the legal right to make the decision regarding continued life support?

a. Patient's mother
b. Patient's 18-year old daughter
c. Patient's estranged husband
d. Facility's ethics committee

17. When developing evidence-based guidelines to reduce urinary tract infections in patients with indwelling catheters, it is important that new policies are based on

a. best practices identified through a literature review.
b. nursing staff preferences.
c. physician preferences.
d. cost-effectiveness.

18. A 25-year-old woman developed classic Guillain-Barré syndrome (acute inflammatory demyelinating polyneuropathy), characterized by rapidly ascending paralysis, progressive weakness, and pain in the buttocks and hips. Which of the following treatments is most appropriate to reduce symptoms and the duration of illness?

a. Corticosteroids
b. Analgesics
c. Intravenous immunoglobulin or plasmapheresis
d. Physical therapy

19. An 18-year-old male patient presents with status epilepticus that has persisted for 15 minutes. Which of the following treatments should the nurse practitioner initiate?

a. Gabapentin, levetiracetam, or topiramate
b. Ethosuximide, valproic acid, or lamotrigine
c. Carbamazepine, oxcarbazepine, or lamotrigine
d. Diazepam, lorazepam, or fosphenytoin

20. A male Hispanic patient is admitted to the unit, and the nurse practitioner is doing the admission history; however, the patient speaks very little English. What should the nurse practitioner do next?

a. Ask the patient's 12-year old son, who is fluent in English, to translate.
b. Use sign language and pictures to supplement questions.
c. Arrange for a translator.
d. Ask the patient's wife, who speaks fair English, to answer the questions for her husband.

21. A patient with a history of narcotics abuse has been taking lorazepam for anxiety but presents with lethargy, dizziness, headache, marked alternations in consciousness, respiratory depression, and ataxia. Her friend states that the patient was found 2 hours earlier with an empty prescription bottle. Which of the following treatments should the nurse practitioner initiate?

a. Gastric emptying and charcoal
b. Charcoal, concentrated dextrose, thiamine, and naloxone
c. Charcoal, concentrated dextrose, and flumazenil
d. Gastric emptying, charcoal, and naloxone

22. A trauma victim has fractures of the upper two ribs on the right side. The patient should be carefully assessed for which secondary injury or injuries?

a. Liver trauma
b. Splenic trauma
c. Tracheal, bronchial, or great vessel trauma
d. Cardiac and splenic trauma

23. A patient recovering from a stroke has persistent dysphagia and is at risk for aspiration. The nurse practitioner should collaborate with which of the following professionals to assess the patient's ability to swallow and to plan therapy?

a. Speech-language pathologist
b. Nutritionist
c. Physical therapist
d. Occupational therapist

24. Ensuring that a patient has given informed consent and understands his or her rights and all of the risks and benefits of a procedure or treatment supports the ethical principal of

a. beneficence.
b. nonmaleficence.
c. justice.
d. autonomy.

25. The nurse practitioner has provided a diabetic patient with literature and videotapes about diabetes and skin care, but the patient has retained little information. However, the patient seems interested in learning and asks many detailed questions. This suggests that the patient's learning style is

a. auditory.
b. kinesthetic.
c. visual.
d. mixed.

26. A patient recovering from abdominal trauma after an automobile accident experiences Abdominal distension, decreased cardiac output, increased respiratory distress, lethargy, and decreased urinary output. Based on these symptoms, which of the following would be most useful for diagnosis?

a. Abdominal x-ray
b. Abdominal ultrasound
c. Abdominal computed tomography
d. Measurement of intra-abdominal pressure

27. The nurse practitioner participates in collaborative activities with others as well as initiating them. Under the Association of Critical Care Nurses' Synergy Model of Collaboration, the nurse is functioning at which level?

a. Level 1
b. Level 2
c. Level 3
d. Level 4

28. When collaborating with other members in team building, which of the following usually occurs during initial interactions?

a. Team members begin to define roles and develop relationships.
b. Team members observe the leader and determine how control is exercised.
c. Team members clarify methods to achieve work.
d. Team members develop rapport, and interactions become less formal.

29. The most common cause of decreased cardiac output after cardiac surgery is

a. persistent bleeding.
b. hypovolemia.
c. bradycardia.
d. cardiac failure.

30. A patient with a cerebral aneurysm dies suddenly on the way to surgery, and the patient's husband shouts at the nurse practitioner, "It is your fault my wife died!" The most appropriate response in this situation is,

a. "There was nothing anyone could do."
b. "She should have come to the hospital sooner."
c. "It is not my fault."
d. "I am so sorry for your loss."

31. A trauma patient exhibits chest pain, pulsus paradoxus, and Beck's triad (i.e., increased central venous pressure with distended neck veins, muffled heart sounds, hypotension). Which of the following interventions is indicated?

a. Angioplasty
b. Pericardiocentesis
c. Transmyocardial revascularization
d. Cardioversion

32. The nurse practitioner is participating in problem-solving using a systems thinking approach to establish new procedures to reduce the incidence of medication and treatment errors. The first step is to

a. describe behavior patterns.
b. define the issue.
c. define patterns of performance and behavior.
d. establish cause–effect relationships.

33. A patient with stage 3 breast cancer states that she feels very hopeful that the treatment will be effective and reports that her friends and family are taking turns providing meals and assisting her. Under the synergy model, which patient characteristic does this reflect?

a. Complexity
b. Stability
c. Vulnerability
d. Resiliency

34. A 55-year-old patient with cryptogenic organizing pneumonitis (formerly bronchiolitis obliterans organizing pneumonia) has developed acute onset of dyspnea, dry cough, low-grade fever, and weight loss. Lung volumes remain normal on x-ray with peripheral and alveolar "ground glass" infiltrates; pulmonary function tests show restriction. Which initial treatment is indicated?

a. Antibiotics
b. Bronchodilators
c. Cytotoxic agents
d. Corticosteroids

35. A 30-year old patient who has had repeated bouts of severe asthmatic attacks tells the nurse practitioner that she has no insurance and cannot afford to take preventive medications. The most appropriate referral is to a

a. free clinic.
b. pharmacy assistance program.
c. social worker.
d. local charitable organization.

36. Which of the following symptoms are consistent with peripheral arterial insufficiency?

a. Pale, shiny, cool skin on the lower extremities
b. Brownish discoloration around the ankles and anterior tibial area
c. Moderate-to-severe peripheral edema
d. Aching and cramping pain

37. The cost-containment committee has decided to limit the types of catheter products to cut costs because of reduced reimbursements by Medicare, Medicaid, and insurance companies. This is an example of the delivery of care impacted by

a. social forces.
b. political forces.
c. regulatory forces.
d. economic forces.

38. Which of the following teaching tools is most effective for patients with low literacy skills?

a. Posters
b. Videos
c. Materials written at a fourth-grade level
d. Slide show presentations

39. When assessing factors that affect readiness to learn, a patient's cultural background and personal goals relate to which of the following?

a. Physical factors
b. Mental/emotional status
c. Experience
d. Knowledge/education

40. According to systems theory (Karl Ludwig von Bertalanffy), the element of a system that comprises actions that take place to transform input is known as

a. throughput.
b. output.
c. evaluation.
d. feedback.

41. When two parties are negotiating informally and make concessions to reach consensus but neither side is really happy with the result, the approach to negotiation is called

a. accommodation.
b. avoidance.
c. compromise.
d. collaboration.

42. When evaluating literature and information to determine the level of evidence, the category that indicates that information has supporting evidence from some studies, has a good theoretical basis, and is strongly recommended for implementation is

a. category IA.
b. category IB.
c. category II.
d. category III.

43. A patient has stage 2 or moderate chronic obstructive pulmonary disease. The primary means of slowing progression of the disease is

a. smoking cessation.
b. pulmonary rehabilitation.
c. bronchodilators.
d. corticosteroids.

44. A violation of professional boundaries is best described of which of the following scenarios?

a. The nurse assists the patient to make a telephone call.
b. The nurse accepts a gift of candy to be shared by all staff members in the unit.
c. The nurse pats the patient's arm to show support.
d. The nurse confides in the patient that she is distressed because her mother is sick.

45. A 65-year-old patient was admitted to the hospital after being found unresponsive. Family members state she had complained of a headache earlier in the day. On admission, her vital signs were as follows:

- Blood pressure: 160/98 mm Hg
- Pulse: 52 beats per minute
- Respirations: 16 breaths per minute
- Temperature: 38°C
- Glasgow coma score: 5

Which of the following imaging studies is the first priority?

a. Head x-ray
b. Head magnetic resonance imaging
c. Head computed tomography (noncontrast)
d. Cerebral angiograms

46. The nurse practitioner is planning classes to educate diabetic patients about monitoring glucose levels. Which educational approach would be most appropriate?

a. One-on-one instruction
b. Educational workshop
c. Lecture
d. Discussion

47. A patient recovering from a craniotomy is on decreasing doses of corticosteroids, but protocol requires 3 more weeks of treatment. Because of the steroid therapy, the patient has developed diabetes insipidus with polydipsia, unrelieved by drinking, and polyuria. Which initial treatment is indicated?

a. Desmopressin acetate, oral or nasal
b. Discontinuation of corticosteroids
c. Indomethacin and hydrochlorothiazide
d. Hydrochlorothiazide

48. A patient with adrenal insufficiency (Addison's disease) has been stable on hydrocortisone and fludrocortisone. However, the patient has been experiencing diarrhea and vomiting and presents with hypotension (86/50 mm Hg), elevated temperature, abdominal pain, and confusion. Which initial intervention is indicated?

a. Laboratory tests for sodium and potassium levels
b. Abdominal computed tomography scan
c. Administration of intravenous hydrocortisone (100 mg) over 30 seconds
d. Administration of fludrocortisone (0.1 mg)

49. Which of the following is an example of therapeutic communication?

a. "You should try not to worry."
b. "Don't worry. Everything will be fine."
c. "Why are you so upset?"
d. "I would like to hear how you feel about that?"

50. When monitoring a patient with a history of ventricular tachycardia, which of the following dysrhythmias is most concerning?

a. Premature atrial contractions
b. Premature ventricular contractions
c. First-degree block
d. Atrial fibrillation with a controlled rate of 110 beats per minute

Answer Key and Explanations

1. C: The total nutrient admixture (TNA) should be discarded if there is "cracking" of the lipid emulsion and the oil separates into a layer. With TNA, all the components of parenteral nutrition and lipids are admixed together in one container to create a 3-in-1 formula. Components of parenteral nutrition generally include proteins, carbohydrates, fats, electrolytes, vitamins, sterile water, and trace vitamins. While most postoperative patients need 1500 calories/day to prevent protein breakdown, those with fever, burns, major surgery, trauma, or hypermetabolic disease may need up to 10,000 calories daily.

2. B: The nurse practitioner should give morphine, as 8 on a 1–10 scale represents severe pain, which is not uncommon in the first 24 hours after surgery. Patients have a right to pain control, and the nurse practitioner should trust that the pain is what the patient says it is. Patients may show very different behavior when they are in pain. Some may cry and moan with minor pain, and others may exhibit little difference in behavior when truly suffering. Thus, judging pain by behavior can lead to the wrong conclusions. Questioning family members is not appropriate.

3. D: The risk of fat embolism syndrome (FES) is greatest with multiple fractures or fractures of the long bones, ribs, or pelvis. Those 20–30 years of age and elderly adults with fractures of the proximal femur are at increased risk. Onset of symptoms (i.e., hypoxia, tachypnea, elevated temperature, tachycardia) is usually at 24–72 hours but may be delayed for up to 7 days.

- Early signs include respiratory alkalosis, progressing to respiratory acidosis and leading to respiratory distress syndrome and congestive heart failure.
- Fat emboli in the brain cause central nervous system abnormalities, such as headache and confusion, leading to coma.
- Systemic embolization may cause widespread petechiae, elevated temperature (> 39.5°C), and kidney failure.

4. A: Patients' rights and autonomy are tied to age, not economics. Regardless of who pays the medical bills, a 19-year-old is an adult by law and can make his own decisions, so his partner must be allowed to visit. The parents do not have a legal right to interfere. The nurse must respect the individual's sexual identification, remain supportive, and should be knowledgeable about issues important to gay, lesbian, bisexual, and transgender patients. The rights and needs of partners should also be respected.

5. B: The treatment of choice for a patient with cirrhosis and refractory ascites awaiting transplant is the transjugular intrahepatic shunt, which involves placing a stent between the hepatic vein and portal circulation. This allows for better excretion of sodium and better response to diuretics. Diuretics are a first-line therapy. Paracentesis is not routinely done except to relieve respiratory distress for those who do not respond adequately to large doses of diuretics and sodium restriction, but relief is temporary as ascites recurs.

6. D: For various reasons, some people may be excluded from a study so that instead of randomized subjects, the subjects may be highly selected; thus, when data, which have internal validity, are compared with another population in which there is more or less selection, results may be different. The selection of subjects, in this case, would interfere with external validity. Part of the design of a study should include considerations of whether or not it should have external validity or whether there is value for the institution based solely on internal validation.

7. C: Nonsteroidal anti-inflammatory drugs (NSAIDs) and corticosteroids are the primary treatments for mild-to-moderate systemic lupus erythematosus (SLE). The NSAIDs are added to the steroids to reduce pain and inflammation and to decrease the steroid dose. SLE is a systemic reaction to collagen or connective tissue in the body; it believed to be triggered by an antibody–antigen immune response to an environmental agent, resulting in widespread damage to vessels and organs, primarily in women. Immunosuppressive agents are

usually reserved for more severe disease if patients do not respond to more conservative treatments. In some cases, antimalarial drugs may be used to control cutaneous or mild SLE.

8. B: Acute lung injury results in severely compromised lungs with crackling rales, wheezing, decreased pulmonary compliance, and cyanosis; thus, oxygen therapy is provided to maintain oxygen saturation over 90%. Oxygen should be administered at 100% because of the mismatch between ventilation and perfusion, which can result in hypoxia on position change. Endotracheal intubation may be needed if oxygen saturation falls or carbon dioxide levels rise.

9. A: Barriers to systems thinking include a reliance on past experience. New directions require new solutions, so being mired in the past or relying solely on past experience can prevent progress. Systems thinking describes having the background knowledge and practical tools to manage both environmental and system resources, within and outside the health care system, to solve problems for the patient and family and meet their needs. Other barriers include the following:

- Feelings of victimization
- Autocratic views
- Identification with role rather than purpose
- Failure to adapt
- Weak consensus

10. C: Laboratory abnormalities consistent with disseminated intravascular coagulation include prolonged prothrombin and partial prothrombin times and decreased platelet count and fibrinogen with fragmented red blood cells. Treatment includes identifying the underlying cause, blood replacement products, anticoagulation therapy to increase clotting time, cryoprecipitate to increase fibrinogen levels, and administration of coagulation inhibitors and coagulation factors.

11. B: Symptoms typical of metabolic alkalosis include elevated serum pH, a relatively normal positive pressure of carbon dioxide (if compensated) or increased (if uncompensated), and a urine pH over 6 (if compensated). The patient is dizzy, confused, and exhibiting tremors, seizures, tingling, tachycardia, arrhythmias. Metabolic alkalosis occurs with decreased strong acid or increased base, with compensatory carbon dioxide retention by the lungs associated with hypoventilation. Metabolic alkalosis is usually caused by excessive vomiting, gastric suctioning, diuretics, potassium deficit, excessive mineralocorticoids, or excessive sodium bicarbonate intake.

12. D: Root-cause analysis is a retrospective attempt to determine the cause of an event, often a sentinel event, such as an unexpected death, or a cluster of events. Root-cause analysis involves interviews, observations, and review of medical records. Often an extensive questionnaire is completed by the person doing the root-cause analysis, tracing essentially every step in hospitalization and care, including every treatment, every medication, and every contact. The focus of the root-cause analysis is on systems and processes rather than individuals.

13. C: The patient described in the question is exhibiting signs of ketoacidosis, so initial treatment includes insulin therapy by continuous infusion, fluid (nonglucose) therapy, and electrolyte replacement. Typical symptoms include Kussmaul respirations (i.e., hyperventilation with "ketone breath" to eliminate carbon dioxide) and fluid imbalance (i.e., loss of potassium and other electrolytes as a result of cellular death), resulting in dehydration from diuresis, excessive thirst, cardiac arrhythmias (i.e., from potassium loss), and hyperglycemia (blood glucose: 300–800 mg/dL).

14. B: The patient described in the question most likely has developed paralytic ileus (i.e., paralysis of the bowel), which can result from infection (e.g., pancreatitis), narcotics, excessive manipulation during surgery, and prolonged anesthesia. Symptoms of bowel obstruction are similar but often more severe with abdominal

rigidity, shock, respiratory distress, and sepsis. Bowel infarction causes acute abdomen and shock. Short gut (bowel) syndrome results from a malabsorptive condition after removal of part of the small intestine.

15. A: Hyperkalemia often occurs with renal disease and is characterized by ventricular arrhythmia, weakness with ascending paralysis and hyperreflexia, diarrhea, and confusion. Hypokalemia is characterized by weakness, lethargy, nausea, vomiting, paresthesias, dysrhythmias (e.g., premature ventricular contractions, flattened T waves), muscle cramps with hyporeflexia, hypotension, and tetany. Hypocalcemia is characterized by tetany, tingling, seizures, altered mental status, and ventricular tachycardia. Hypercalcemia is characterized by increasing muscle weakness with hypotonicity, constipation, anorexia, nausea, vomiting, and bradycardia.

16. C: The patient's estranged husband has a health care power of attorney, which gives him the right to make decisions if the patient is unable to do so. While divorce may automatically revoke the health care power of attorney in some states, the patient and her husband are not divorced. The legal document takes precedence over family ties, such as those of the mother and daughter. This is not a decision rendered by an ethics committee. If family members want to challenge the husband, their recourse is to take the matter to court.

17. A: While all of the elements listed in the question are important, best practices identified through literature review should carry the most weight when developing evidence-based guidelines. Preferences are often based on subjective observations rather than objective observations and may relate to familiarity and ease of use. Cost-effectiveness is always an issue and must be considered, but it should not be the primary concern. In some cases, spending more to prevent a problem initially may save money in terms of morbidity and extended medical care in the long term.

18. C: Intravenous immunoglobulin (IVIg) and plasmapheresis are the only treatments that have been proven to be effective for Guillain-Barré syndrome, which is a group of immune disorders, primarily involving the peripheral nervous system and resulting in paralysis and weakness. IVIg tends to have fewer complications and is easier to use than plasmapheresis; there is no advantage in combining the two treatments. Corticosteroids do not have an effect on the disease's progress. Analgesics may be used to maintain comfort, but they are not the primary treatment. Physical therapy may be useful after the acute stage of the disease if the patient has residual weakness.

19. D: Status epilepticus is treated with benzodiazepines, such as diazepam, lorazepam, or fosphenytoin. Phenytoin and phenobarbital are used if there is no response from a benzodiazepine. A patent airway must be established (i.e., jaw thrust may reduce obstruction from muscle rigidity). An intravenous line must be established, and electrolytes, blood gases, and glucose levels are monitored with glucose administration for hypoglycemia. A nasogastric tube may be inserted. Generalized seizures are treated with gabapentin, levetiracetam, or topiramate. Absence seizures are treated with ethosuximide, valproic acid, or lamotrigine. Partial seizures are treated with carbamazepine, oxcarbazepine, or lamotrigine.

20. C: The nurse should arrange for a translator. Children should never be used as translators as they lack the vocabulary and understanding about health matters and may not interpret correctly. Other adult family members, such as the wife, should not be asked to answer questions for the patient unless the patient is unable to answer questions because of a health condition because they may not understand medical terms and may not translate correctly. Additionally, the patient may have kept information from the family.

21. B: Because the patient has been taking lorazepam and has a history of narcotic use, the nurse practitioner should suspect co-ingestion, especially since the patient is exhibiting alternations in consciousness and respiratory depression. In this case charcoal, concentrated dextrose, thiamine, and naloxone are indicated. Gastric emptying is indicated only if ingestion occurred less than 1 hour ago. Flumazenil (antagonist), 0.2 mg each minute to a total of 3 mg, may be used in some cases but is not routinely advised because of complications related to benzodiazepine dependency or co-ingestion of cyclic antidepressants. Flumazenil is contraindicated in the presence of increased intracranial pressure.

22. C: Underlying injuries should be expected, according to the area of fractures:

- Upper 2 ribs: injury to the trachea, bronchi, or great vessels
- Right-sided rib 8 or above: trauma to the liver
- Left-sided rib 8 or above: trauma to the spleen

Pain, often localized or experienced on respirations or compression of the chest, may be the primary symptom of rib fractures, resulting in shallow breathing that can lead to atelectasis or pneumonia. Fractured ribs are usually the result of severe trauma, such as blunt force from a motor vehicle accident or physical abuse.

23. A: The stroke patient should be evaluated by a speech-language pathologist, who can evaluate muscle activity, assess speech, and assess memory to determine the extent of pathology associated with the dysphagia. The pathologist may recommend certain types of foods, such as thickened liquids, to decrease the chance of aspiration. A referral may then be made to a physical therapist to help the patient strengthen weak muscles and learn strategies, such as sitting upright and using a straw for fluids, to decrease dysphagia.

24. D: Autonomy is the ethical principle that ensures the individual has the right to make decisions about his or her own care. The nurse practitioner must keep patients fully informed so they can exercise autonomy in informed decision-making. Beneficence is an ethical principle that involves performing actions that benefit another person. Nonmaleficence is an ethical principle that ensures health care workers provide care in a manner that does not cause intentional harm to the patient. Justice is the ethical principle that relates to the distribution of the limited resources of health care benefits to members of society.

25. A: The patient's learning style is auditory. While learning style does vary some from person to person, all people learn from visual information, auditory information, and by hands-on learning. In general, the best practice would be to apply a mixture of materials when addressing any patient.

Auditory learners	Learn best by listening and talking: Explain procedures while demonstrating, and have the learner repeat. Plan extra time to discuss and answer questions. Provide audiotapes.
Visual learners	Learn best by seeing and reading: Provide written directions and picture guides, or demonstrate procedures. Use charts and diagrams. Provide photos or videos.
Kinesthetic learners	Learn best by handling, doing, and practicing: Provide hands-on experience throughout teaching. Encourage handling of supplies and equipment. Allow the learner to demonstrate. Minimize instructions, and allow the person to explore equipment and procedures.

26. D: The symptoms listed in the question (i.e., abdominal distension, decreased cardiac output, increased respiratory distress, lethargy, decreased urinary output) are consistent with compartment syndrome. Diagnosis of abdominal compartment syndrome is by measurement of intra-abdominal pressure (> 25 cm H_2O) by a Foley catheter or a nasogastric tube with a pressure transducer or water-column manometry. Abdominal trauma with pronounced shock increases the risk of compartment syndrome. Pressure within the abdomen may begin to rise rapidly if the abdomen is closed, resulting in decreased cardiac output from pressure on the vena cava; increased airway pressures and acute respiratory distress syndrome; decreased urinary output with a decrease in renal blood flow and glomerular filtration; increased central venous pressure, resulting in increased intracranial pressure; and cerebral edema.

27. B: The nurse is functioning at level 2 of 3. There is no level 4.

- Level 1: This nurse participates in collaborative activities, learns from others, including mentors, and respects the input of others.
- Level 2: This nurse not only participates in collaborative activities but also initiates them and actively seeks learning opportunities.
- Level 3: This nurse takes a leadership role in collaborative activities by mentoring and teaching others while still seeking learning opportunities and actively seeking resources as needed.

28. A: Members begin to define their roles and develop relationships in their initial interactions.

- Power issues: Members observe the leader and determine who controls the meetings and how control is exercised; they begin to form alliances.
- Organizing: Members clarify methods to achieve work and begin to work together, gaining respect for each other's contributions and working toward a common goal.
- Team identification: Members develop rapport, and interactions often become less formal as members help and support each other to achieve goals.
- Excellence: Good leadership, committed team members, clear goals, high standards, external recognition, spirit of collaboration, and a shared commitment to the process lead to excellence.

29. B: Hypovolemia is the most common cause of decreased cardiac output after cardiac surgery. Hypovolemia may result from a net loss of fluids during surgery as well as fluid shift into the third space because of increased permeability of capillaries. Hypothermia may also contribute to hypovolemia because the blood vessels dilate, requiring more blood, as the body temperature increases during rewarming. Tachydysrhythmias are more common after surgery than bradydysrhythmias, although pacing wires may be left in place to stimulate the heart. Bloody discharge should be measured carefully and should not exceed 200 mL/hr for 4–6 hours after surgery.

30. D: The most appropriate response is, "I'm so sorry for your loss." Trying to deflect blame to the patient or others or make excuses serves little purpose. Elisabeth Kübler-Ross identified five stages of grief in *On Death and Dying* (1969), which can apply to both patients and family members: denial, anger, bargaining, depression, and acceptance. Patients and families often react with pronounced anger, directed inwardly or outwardly. Women often blame themselves because of some personal action, and self-anger often leads to severe depression and guilt. Outward anger is more common in men and may be expressed as overt hostility.

31. B: Beck's triad is an indication of cardiac tamponade, treated with pericardiocentesis with a large bore needle or surgical repair to control bleeding and relieve cardiac compression. Cardiac tamponade occurs with pericardial effusion in which fluid accumulates in the pericardial sac, causing pressure against the heart. It may be a complication of trauma, pericarditis, cardiac surgery, or heart failure. Other symptoms may include a feeling of pressure or pain in the chest and dyspnea, and pulsus paradoxus (i.e., systolic blood pressure heard during exhalation but not during inhalation) over 10 mm Hg may be present.

32. B: The first step is to define the issue by describing the problem in detail without judgment or solutions. Other steps include:

- Describe behavior patterns: List factors related to the problem, using graphs to outline possible trends.
- Establish cause–effect relationships: Use the "Five Whys" or other
- root-cause analysis and feedback loops.
- Define patterns of performance and behavior: Determine how variables affect outcomes and the types of patterns of behavior currently taking place.
- Find solutions: Discuss possible solutions and outcomes.
- Institute performance improvement activities: Make changes, and then monitor for changes in behavior.

33. D: Resiliency is the ability to recover from a devastating illness and regain a sense of stability, both physically and emotionally. Supporting factors include faith, a positive sense of hope, and a supportive network of friends and family. Complexity occurs when more than one system is involved: internal (e.g., cardiac and renal systems) or external (e.g., addicted and homeless) or some combination (e.g., ill with poor family dynamics). Stability allows a person to maintain a state of physical and emotional equilibrium despite illness and challenges. Vulnerability includes factors (e.g., anxiety, fear, prejudice, lack of information) that put a person at increased risk and interfere with recovery and compliance.

34. D: Corticosteroids successfully treat about three-quarters of cases of cryptogenic organizing pneumonitis (COP). Prognosis is good if the patient responds well to treatment, although relapses may occur. Bronchiolitis is inflammation of the bronchioles and may be constrictive, such as from scarring caused by chronic inflammation, or proliferative, in which exudate obstructs the bronchiole lumen, resulting in cough. With bronchiolitis obliterans/COP the exudate invades the alveolar spaces, increasing dyspnea. COP is most common in adults between 50 and 60 years of age.

35. C: The most appropriate referral for a patient with no insurance and an inability to buy medications is to a social worker who can evaluate the patient's needs and income to determine for what, if any, programs the patient may be eligible. Free clinics and charitable organizations may not be able to provide for ongoing medical needs. The social worker can assess eligibility for pharmacy assistance plans, which may vary, but most require income of less than 200% of the federal poverty level.

36. A: Pale, shiny, cool skin on the lower extremities is consistent with peripheral arterial insufficiency.

Characteristic	Arterial Insufficiency	Venous Insufficiency
Pain	Ranges from intermittent claudication to severe and constant	Aching/cramping
Pulses	Weak or absent	Present
Skin	Rubor on dependency but pallor of foot on elevation Pale, shiny, cool skin with loss of hair on toes and foot Thick and ridged nails	Brownish discoloration around ankles and anterior tibial area
Ulcers	Painful, deep, circular, often necrotic ulcers on toe tips, toe webs, heels, or other pressure areas	Varying degrees of pain in superficial, irregular ulcers on medial or lateral malleolus and sometimes the anterior tibial area
Edema	Minimal	Moderate to severe

37. D: Economic forces, such as managed care or cost-containment committees, try to contain costs to insurers and facilities by controlling access to and duration of treatment and limiting products. Social forces, such as increased demand for access to treatment and medical services, include both traditional and complementary medicine. Political forces affect medical care as the federal and state governments increasingly become purchasers of medical care, imposing their guidelines and limitations on the medical system. Regulatory forces, which may be local, state, or federal, can have a profound effect on delivery of care and services, differing from one state or region to another.

38. B: Videos are more effective than written materials for those with low literacy or poor English skills. Focused viewing in which the nurse discusses the purpose of the video presentation before viewing and then is available for discussion after viewing can be very effective. Patients and families are often nervous about learning patient care and are unsure of their abilities. Allowing the patients and families to watch a video demonstration or explanation first and allowing them to stop or review the video presentation can help them to grasp the fundamentals before they have to apply them.

39. C: People's experience with learning can vary widely and is affected by their ability to cope with changes, their personal goals, motivation to learn, and cultural background. People may have widely divergent ideas about what constitutes illness and treatment. Lack of English skills may make learning difficult and prevent people from asking questions. Readiness to learn should be assessed because if patients and families are not ready, instruction is of little value. Often readiness is indicated when the patients and families ask questions or show an interest in procedures.

40. A: Karl Ludwig von Bertalanffy believed that all of the elements of a system interact to achieve goals, and a change in any one element will impact the other elements and alter outcomes. The five elements in a system include the following:

- Input: This is what goes into a system in terms of energy or materials.
- Throughput: These are the actions that take place to transform input.
- Output: This is the result of the interrelationship between input and processes.
- Evaluation: This is the process of monitoring success or failure.
- Feedback: This is information that results from the process and can be used to evaluate the end result.

41. C: The different approaches to negotiation follow:

Compromise	Both parties make concessions, but this can result in decisions that suit no one; thus, compromise is not always ideal.
Accommodation	One party concedes to the other, but the losing side may gain little or nothing; thus, this approach should be used when there is clear benefit to one choice.
Avoidance	When both parties dislike conflict, they may put off negotiating and resolve nothing.
Collaboration	Both parties receive what they want, often through creative solutions, but collaboration may be ineffective with highly competitive parties.
Competition	One party wins and the other loses, sometimes resulting in conflict.

42. B: The category that indicates that information has supporting evidence from some studies, has a good theoretical basis, and is strongly recommended for implementation is category IB. A list of categories include the following:

- Category IA: Information is well supported by evidence from experimental, clinical, or epidemiological studies and is strongly recommended for implementation.
- Category IB: Information has supporting evidence from some studies, a good theoretical basis, and is strongly recommended for implementation.
- Category IC: Information is required by state or federal regulations or an industry standard
- Category II: Information is supported by suggestive clinical or epidemiologic studies, has a theoretical basis, and is suggested for implementation.
- Category III: Information is supported by descriptive studies and may be useful.
- Category IV: Information is obtained from expert opinion or authorities only.
- Unresolved: No information is recommended because of a lack of consensus or evidence.

43. A: Smoking cessation is the primary means of slowing the progression of chronic obstructive pulmonary disease and may require smoking cessation support in the form of classes or medications, such as bupropion, nicotine patches or gum, clonidine, or nortriptyline. Pulmonary rehabilitation includes breathing exercises, muscle training, activity pacing, and modification of activities to reduce symptoms. Bronchodilators, such as albuterol and salmeterol, relieve bronchospasm and airway obstruction. Corticosteroids, both inhaled and oral (prednisone), may improve symptoms but are used most often for associated asthma.

44. D: The nurse must respect and maintain the confidentiality of the patient and family members, but the nurse must also be very careful about disclosing personal information because this establishes a social relationship that interferes with professional boundaries. The nurse and patient should never share "secrets."

When the nurse divulges personal information, he or she may become vulnerable to the patient, which is a reversal of roles.

45. C: Noncontrast head computed tomography (CT) should be done to differentiate between cerebral infarct and cerebral hemorrhage. CT is more effective than magnetic resonance imaging (MRI) in detecting cerebral hemorrhage and the extent of a hematoma in the first 48 hours, although it does not always distinguish between an infarct and a tumor. Head x-ray does not provide adequate information. Cerebral angiograms or magnetic resonance angiography may be completed after CT in some cases to determine if an aneurysm or arteriovenous malformation is present.

46. B: Educational workshops are usually conducted with small groups, allowing for maximal participation, and are especially good for demonstrations and practice sessions, such as for patients learning to monitor glucose levels. One-on-one instruction is helpful for targeted instruction in procedures for individuals, but it is time-intensive and less cost-effective. Lectures are often used for academic or detailed information and may include time for questions and answers, but discussions are limited. Discussions are best with small groups so that people can actively participate; they are a good for problem-solving.

47. A: Desmopressin acetate is the treatment of choice for steroid-induced diabetes insipidus. Corticosteroids cannot be abruptly discontinued, although the condition should improve as the doses decrease. Central and nephrogenic diabetes insipidus may respond to hydrochlorothiazide, and nephrogenic diabetes insipidus may respond to combined therapy. Diabetes insipidus is caused by a deficiency of the antidiuretic hormone (ADH), or vasopressin. Diabetes insipidus may develop secondary to head trauma, primary brain tumor, meningitis, encephalitis, corticosteroid therapy, surgical ablation or irradiation of the pituitary, or metastatic tumors. In congenital nephrogenic diabetes insipidus, production of ADH is normal, but the renal tubules do not respond.

48. C: Because the symptoms listed in the question (i.e., diarrhea, vomiting, hypotension, elevated temperature, abdominal pain, confusion) are consistent with an adrenal crisis, which is life-threatening, treatment with hydrocortisone (usually 100 mg) intravenously over 30 seconds should be provided immediately without waiting for confirming laboratory tests. Hyponatremia and hyperkalemia are common findings. Adrenal crisis often presents with symptoms similar to acute abdomen and may be precipitated by gastrointestinal infections or other stressors. Following the bolus of hydrocortisone, large-volume infusions of saline solution are provided until dehydration, hypotension, and hyponatremia are corrected. Hydrocortisone administration continues with decreasing steroid doses over three 24-hour periods. Fludrocortisone is provided after intravenous saline treatment is completed.

49. D: "I would like to hear how you feel about that" is an example of therapeutic communication that allows a patient to explore a topic. Examples of nontherapeutic communication include the following:

- Meaningless clichés: "Don't worry. Everything will be fine." "Isn't it a nice day?"
- Providing advice: "You should...." "The best thing to do is...." When patients ask for advice, it is better to provide facts and encourage the patient to reach a decision.
- Asking for explanations of behavior not directly related to patient care: "Why are you upset?"

50. B: Premature ventricular contractions (PVCs) are of most concern for a patient with a history of ventricular tachycardia (VT) because they may indicate the onset of more serious and life-threatening dysrhythmias. Recurrent PVCs can lead to VT. In general, premature atrial contractions (PACs), atrial fibrillation, (controlled rate), and first-degree atrioventricular (AV) block are less pathological than VT, ventricular fibrillation, asystole, and second-degree and third-degree AV blocks. In patients without a history of heart disease, PVCs and skipped beats are of less concern and usually require no treatment other than ensuring correct electrolyte balance and avoiding caffeine.

Online Resources

Due to our efforts to try to keep this book to a manageable length, we've created a link that will give you access to all of your online resources:

mometrix.com/resources719/acnpc

It's Your Moment, Let's Celebrate It!

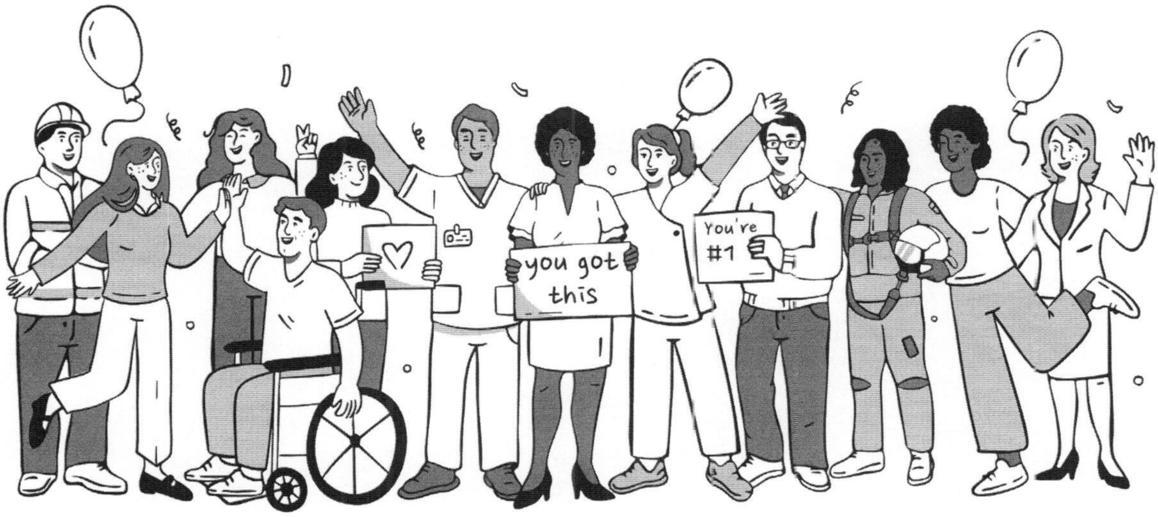

Share your story @mometrixtestpreparation